Cultivating Qi

of related interest

Vital Breath of the Dao
Chinese Shamanic Tiger Qigong—Laohu Gong
Master Zhongxian Wu
ISBN 978 1 84819 000 9
eISBN 978 0 85701 110 7

Daoist Nei Gong
The Philosophical Art of Change
Damo Mitchell
Foreword by Cindy Engel
ISBN 978 1 84819 065 8
eISBN 978 0 85701 033 9

Qigong Through the Seasons
How to Stay Healthy All Year with Qigong,
Meditation, Diet, and Herbs
Ronald H. Davis
Illustrated by Pamm Davis
Foreword by Ken Cohen
ISBN 978 1 84819 238 6
eISBN 978 0 85701 185 5

The Way of the Five Seasons
Living with the Five Elements for Physical,
Emotional, and Spiritual Harmony
John Kirkwood
ISBN 978 1 84819 301 7
eISBN 978 0 85701 252 4

Cultivating
Qi

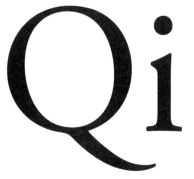

The Root of Energy, Vitality, and Spirit

David W. Clippinger
Foreword by Grandmaster Nick Gracenin

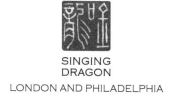

SINGING
DRAGON

LONDON AND PHILADELPHIA

First published in 2016
by Singing Dragon
an imprint of Jessica Kingsley Publishers
73 Collier Street
London N1 9BE, UK
and
400 Market Street, Suite 400
Philadelphia, PA 19106, USA

www.singingdragon.com

Copyright © David W. Clippinger 2016
Foreword copyright © Grandmaster Nick Gracenin 2016

Library of Congress Cataloging in Publication Data
A CIP catalog record for this book is available from the Library of Congress.

British Library Cataloguing in Publication Data
A CIP catalogue record for this book is available from the British Library.

ISBN 978 1 84819 291 1
eISBN 978 0 85701 254 8

Printed and bound in Great Britain

For Philip and Tess
In hopes that these words will keep you
on your own paths of fulfillment

Contents

Foreword

When I began martial arts training in the 1960s, almost no information on the subject was available. During the 1970s, books and magazines, super-8 movies, feature films, and television shows introduced us to the mysterious movements and exotic culture of Asian martial arts. Subsequent decades gave us a flood of information on VHS, DVD, and now e-pubs and digital downloads. YouTube and Vimeo are the teachers of a new generation of martial artists. The mysteries, it would seem, are readily available. Perhaps all but one: Qi.

When Dr. David Clippinger shared with me his intention to write a book about Qi and Qigong, I strongly encouraged the endeavor. While some wonderful material is available on the subject, more is certainly needed. An experienced author with a strong background in academia, Dr. Clippinger is a long-time martial artist and a dedicated teacher. His writing presents not only traditional concepts and directives from past masters, but also his own insights and realizations from many years of experience. *Cultivating Qi* will surely be a welcome addition in the libraries of novices and experts alike.

I have known David for many years. I am pleased to have worked with him on many levels at various martial arts events. He is a valued colleague, dedicated student, fellow teacher and promoter, and a dear friend. I congratulate him on the publication of this new book, and I look forward to future works.

GRANDMASTER NICK GRACENIN
WASHINGTON, DC
NOVEMBER 2015

Acknowledgments

Authors write the books that they would like to read. To paraphrase the American novelist Toni Morrison, if the book that we want to read does not exist yet, we have an obligation to write it. I have spent twenty years looking for a book that bridges Eastern philosophy, Traditional Chinese Medicine, spirituality, and the practice of Internal Martial Arts, and if I have somehow overlooked just such a book during my quest, I apologize, but to date, my search has led to my coming up empty-handed or at best unsatisfied. I have written this book as my foray into creating such a bridge and an attempt to quench my own desire to link theory and practice, philosophy and living, and Qi and Shen.

Any book, including this one, does not come into being without precedents, and many other texts and books and people have helped to bring forth this work. I am indebted to the scholars that have paved the way for me, and two in particular are absolutely vital: Thomas Cleary and his magnificent translations of so many crucial works of Eastern philosophy and religion; and Holmes Welch, with whom I share a spiritual Ch'an lineage and whose works on Taoism and Ch'an Buddhism remain unsurpassed in my eyes.

I am also indebted to many of the masters and grandmasters with whom I have had the opportunity to study—either through seminars, workshops, and group classes, or through individual coaching—including Grandmaster Helen Wu, who has been so central in showing me how the practices of Internal Arts are life itself; Grandmaster Nick Gracenin, who so graciously agreed to write the foreword for this book, and whom I admire and model my own training after so that at some point in the future my practice might reach where his is (although he is always moving ahead of me and I will never catch up to his ever expanding mastery); Dr. Yang, Jwing-Ming; Grandmaster William C.C. Chen; Grandmaster Li Deyin; Dr. Daniel Lee; Master Yang Yang; Grandmaster Xiaoxing Chen; and others. When I read over my own book I can hear many of these wonderful teachers' voices and sayings, and I am indebted to the generosity and grace with which these incredible teachers have shared their wisdom and understanding. I am humbled to claim the book as written by me since I learned so much from each of them, and their voices are interwoven with many of my sentences.

My students over the many years have heard me talk about the ideas of "Song" (being at ease, or relaxation), Structure, and Rooting that are at the heart of *Cultivating Qi*, and they have endured my telling them to relax, root, and align their bodies over and over until they probably have grown weary of it. All of those students—past and present—provided me with the energy to continue with this project and write what proved to be difficult to get into words. (Perhaps that is why this book hadn't been written before, and although other writers simply *recognized* this fact, I was too stubborn to let go!) Those students encouraged me to continue in the face of this difficulty, and for those words of encouragement and support, I am very grateful.

All of my students are dear to me, but I am indebted especially to my senior student Jesse Prentiss, who talked with me ceaselessly over the years about these ideas and who read the manuscript and offered suggestions. Jesse has been more than my student; he has been a true friend for many years and has helped me immensely in ways that transcend just shaping the ideas of this book.

Anita Prentiss, Jesse's wife and a fabulous photographer, deserves recognition for the fine photos throughout the book. Anita's photography studio, Buzzy Photography in Pittsburgh, Pennsylvania, is a remarkable place, and she is an exceptional photographer, artist, and person. I admire her photography, and the depths of her compassionate and positive attitude toward other people and life is readily apparent in every photo she takes.

All of the illustrations have been done by Jane Dudley, who was also the designer of the Still Mountain logo for my T'ai Chi and Chi Kung school. I have been lucky to have someone as talented as Jane do the illustrations, but what is most apropos is that Jane has studied Taiji for many years *and* she is also a Ch'an Buddhist lay monk. Jane's understanding of the Internal Arts coupled with her spiritual background were invaluable in developing illustrations that render the ideas of the book clearly and succinctly. Her creativity, passionate dedication, and tireless effort are deeply appreciated. Those illustrations are a reflection of the depth of her understanding.

This book would not have been possible without my wife Annabelle, who encouraged me when I decided to leave behind a university career and pursue the Internal Arts full time. She has been my biggest supporter for nearly twenty-five years. I am grateful to share my life with her, and without her support, this book and the life behind this book would not be possible.

My son Philip and my daughter Tess are also at the heart of this book. When I was having a difficult time imagining an audience for the book and how I should approach it, I thought of what I would like to say to each of them to help them continue on their own paths. The book is a conversation that I am having with them— encouraging them to grow, search, cultivate, and become more and more human.

Finally, I thank Jessica Kingsley as well as the editors and administrative staff at Singing Dragon for providing me with this opportunity for these ideas to reach others. I am delighted to not only have the support to bring the ideas of this book into print, but also to find myself published alongside so many other exceptional writers, thinkers, and teachers that are part of Singing Dragon's remarkable catalogue of authors.

I hope that others will find that my efforts to create a bridge between theory and practice, ideas and living, have not been in vain.

Introduction

Qi has been an "open secret" for thousands of years, and the material in these pages is not merely my own invention, but is part of a rich and profound lineage of Taoist, Buddhist, and Traditional Chinese Medicine philosophy and practice. But as an "open secret," examples of how Qi impacts the act of living are scarce. The first chapter, "The Will to Qi," explores the fundamentals of Qi and how it relates to both mind and body in the effort to construct a life of value. The chapter recasts the principles and theories of Taoism, Buddhism, and Traditional Chinese Medicine in a more contemporary light to show how Qi is just as vital now as it has been for thousands of years.

The sustained lineage of Qi is the focus of "Returning to the Source: The History of Energy and Its Uses," the second chapter, which details the fundamental principles of Traditional Chinese Medicine—the energetic channels of the body and the Five Elements Theory of the Organs—as well as Taoism, Buddhism, and how each of those practices use Qi for developing health, well-being, awareness, and as a tool for awakening (or enlightenment). The chapter charts the principles of Qi, Jing, and Shen, and the three internal harmonies (body, mind [Yi], and heart [Xin]), which are a necessary context for understanding how Qi is used in the five regulations of classic Taiji training:

1. regulating body

2. regulating breath

3. regulating mind

4. regulating Qi

5. regulating spirit.

"Returning to the Source" provides the backdrop for the remaining chapters that focus on the body, breath, and mind, and how those three elements are an absolute necessity in the development of Qi and spirit.

The body is the foundation of Qi—its literal and physical causeway—and is the most appropriate and accessible starting point for cultivating energy. "Opening the Energy Gates of the Body," the third chapter, builds upon the principles of relaxation—called "Song" (being at ease) in Chinese—as well as the way in which the body processes, uses, and stores energy. This fundamental body principle creates internal harmony, which is then harnessed for the harmony of mind and heart. In this way, body awareness opens the door to the heart and mind (Xin and Yi) and by extension one's relationship to the world at large and its processes. With this understanding, the body becomes a vehicle for recognizing spiritual cultivation and is the access point for actualizing the Tao or "Buddha mind."

Body work of this kind not only paves the way for spiritual cultivation, but is also a gateway to the practice of energetic breath work. Breath is a sacred vehicle in many religions, and it is a fundamental tool for meditation as well as relaxation. The ideogram for Qi includes breath (air), which is a vital component of energy cultivation. The fourth chapter, "Powered by Breath," focuses on techniques such as Buddhist and Taoist (abdominal and reverse abdominal) breathing for the cultivation of energy and how those techniques can be harnessed to enhance body practices. The breath forms a bridge between body and mind and generates a richer sense of harmony. These techniques rest upon the foundation of Song and yield deeper insights into our internal landscape.

Buddhism calls the heart of that internal landscape the fundamental Buddha nature or Buddha mind. In Taoism, it is the original essence (Tao). Whereas the body and breath constitute the soil and proper nutrients for the growth of awareness, insight, and energy, the mind and its consciousness (Shen) is the pivot between oneself and the world. "Cultivating Mind and Heart," Chapter 5, explores traditional approaches to training the mind such as meditation and Internal Arts practices—and how those techniques can be translated into interpersonal dynamics, self-awareness, and a more balanced approach to living. The mind is the bridge between our own internal landscape and the world at large, and these techniques generate a more balanced approach to the individual's internal and external world. With a calm and focused mind, Qi can be cultivated more efficiently for use along the path of discovery.

The approach to working with Qi through the body, breath, and mind can be condensed into three principles that recur throughout each of the chapters: Relaxation, Structure, and Rooting. The quality and flow of Qi depends on the state of the body, breath, and mind, and if each is soft and relaxed, the Qi is smooth and harmonious. Structure translates into how the body is positioned, the method of breathing, and the techniques of cultivating awareness and concentration in the mind, which allows for Qi to be harnessed and circulated. And rooting pertains to establishing the foundation of the body, with the breath flowing smoothly and without obstruction through the body, and the mind penetrating deeply to perceive both internal and external landscapes of the self and the world, allowing for the refinement of Qi and its transformation into Shen (spirit).

The precarious danger in proposing the act of unearthing a more "fulfilling life" is approaching the subject too abstractly (relying upon theoretical, esoteric discussions from various sources that make promises of "enlightenment" but little guidance on how to get there) or too programmatically (a manual of steps that mean if you do these "X" things you too will discover joy and success). This book attempts to balance these two extremes by offering a detailed overview of the philosophies and practices (the "esoteric" context) in Chapter 6, "The Elements of Daily Practice," which offers instruction on a number of methodologies that draw upon a range of sources: seated Ch'an (Buddhist) Meditation; Taoist Standing Meditation; ways of opening the energy gates of the body for Qi flow from Neigong practices; strategies for cultivating Qi in the body from Qigong, Baguaquan, and Taiji; and a Qigong set developed for my students and practiced for many years. This book is a way of discovering oneself, and since no two lives are exactly the same, it avoids being prescriptive since any discoveries are the individual's own and cannot be anticipated. Chapter 6 reframes the philosophical discussions with specific techniques and practices that actualize the concepts thereby bringing these ideas into action through six carefully described practices. These exercises include time-tested ancient methods as well as contemporary, up-to-date techniques, and are presented in clear language accompanied by photos and illustrations. The techniques include:

- Wuji, the famous Taoist version of Standing Meditation

- Kaimen, the ancient Taoist technique of circulating Qi through the body

- Jing Shan Qigong, a Qigong set that integrates all of the principles of this book

- Seated Single-Pointed Meditation (Yi Shou), the standard form of Ch'an (Chinese) Buddhist Meditation

- Reflective Meditation, a directed meditation to gain insight into oneself and others

- Life Applications, a method of assessing Qi and making adjustments as necessary.

One of the most famous Chinese sayings in Taiji training can be translated loosely as "The teacher will lead you to the door, but it is up to the student to improve." My desire is that this book opens a door into a deeper sense of harmony, balance, and peace. And even though Will cannot be taught, I hope that a spark of inspiration crosses over and helps to illuminate the pathway to wholeness. As Lao Tzu writes, "A journey of a thousand miles begins with a single step." My wish is that this book be a useful guide and companion for that journey.

CHAPTER I

The Will to Qi

The multiple lanes of cars and trucks were snarled heading into the tunnel, and many of the drivers appeared to be irritated, angered, bothered, or blank. Just on the other side of the tunnel was a beautiful vista of three different rivers coming together with numerous bridges punctuating the view of the shimmering downtown skyline of Pittsburgh, Pennsylvania. When I drove Grandmaster Helen Wu through the tunnel and we emerged on the other side, she exclaimed, "How beautiful! It reminds me of Shanghai, my hometown, with all of its bridges." The contrast between these two sides of the tunnel was as if the tunnel was the barrier between two very different worlds: one side, a world of metal cars and discontent people aggressively jockeying for position; and the other, a landscape where both the water and the traffic flowed unimpeded.

When my son and daughter were young and we would witness such a traffic snarl and the people aggressively changing lanes or not paying attention, inevitably one of my children would say, "That person isn't being careful," and the other would say, "I hope he or she is okay." Of course, the downside to teaching this awareness is that at any moment my children were more than willing to point out when my driving or any other behavior was less than appropriate, and then they would assume the roles of mini-therapists: "Is everything okay? Are there things bothering you, Dad?" Our actions, thoughts, and words, at every moment, are a direct manifestation of how we are feeling. Our anger, anxiety, stress, and sadness are embedded in our actions. *The Dhammapada*, one of the cornerstones of Buddhist thought and practice, states quite simply that, "We are what we think. All that we are arises with our thoughts. With our thoughts we make the world" (Byrom 1993, p.1). In other words, the world that we live in and the one to which we are reacting is the outward form of our own inward state. If that is indeed the case, we might start worrying about the people who inhabit our modern world; or perhaps, more appropriately, we should worry about ourselves.

The precarious state of the world isn't only a modern problem; it has been with us for quite some time. Over 150 years ago Henry David Thoreau, the American naturalist and philosopher, famously proclaimed that "the mass of men lead lives of quiet desperation. What is called resignation is confirmed desperation" (Sayre 1985, p.329). While Thoreau's statement may seem "contemporary," it illustrates a core human issue: the lack of integration and sense of dissatisfaction we as human beings often feel in our lives. The era of social media has made this despair more pronounced since people now publicly and loudly announce their unhappiness, dissatisfaction, anger, and depression. Despair is no longer quiet. Yet this is not merely a contemporary issue even if the technologies by which those announcements are made are modern.

Evidence of this desperation also can be found at least 2500 years ago. *Lieh Tzu*, a book attributed to Lie Yukou, a Taoist master of the fourth century BCE, reveals a similar condition through one of the tales, "The Man Who Wanted to Forget," which I translate and retell:

> A man by the name of Hua Zi was a successful businessman and head of a prominent household. He began to become more and more forgetful until he seemed completely (yet blissfully) unaware of everything.
>
> His family was distraught by his condition, even though Hua Zi did not seem unhappy in the least. They sought out doctors, healers, and sorcerers to help to heal the man. None were successful until a philosopher agreed to tackle the problem.
>
> Over time, the man gradually began to return to his former self, but when he fully returned, the man grew irate and chased his own family members from the house and then grabbed a hunting spear with the intent of killing the philosopher who had "cured" him. The police restrained the man before he was able to harm the philosopher.

When Hua Zi was questioned about why he went into a murderous rage, he explained that "When I lost my mind, I was happy, carefree, and boundless. Now that I have my mind back, all of my old problems and responsibilities have come flooding back to haunt me. When I forgot myself, I was happy, safe, and serene. Now that my mind is back, I am miserable."

Lie Yukou and Thoreau share the view that the responsibilities of living may seem like a prison from which there is no escape, and our conditioned state, which we think that we must occupy, is one of despair, disease, or even insanity.

Pressure and stress are inevitable. It was such pressure that prompted Thoreau to retreat to the woods by himself to "live deliberately, to front only the essential facts of life" (Sayre 1985, p.394). And it was that same pressure that made Hua Zi, the man who wanted to forget, retreat into madness. The problem is, quite simply, we lose sight of our center as the list of responsibilities grows. Our lives are pulled in different directions, and the various roles, responsibilities asked of us, and our own values become more askew. We even seem to lose the cohesive force that keeps our lives integrated and which provides a sense of value and purpose to our day-to-day existence.

When everything is in balance (Figure 1.1), there is greater congruency within the various aspects of our lives, and a unified sense of purpose balances the various roles and responsibilities that are required of us. Such congruency generates a feeling of satisfaction, harmony, or even joy.

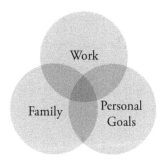

FIGURE I.I A BALANCED LIFE

Yet when responsibilities grow too extreme in one part of our life, the area of overlap shrinks and our focus shifts toward one particular facet, tilting the balance precariously (Figure 1.2).

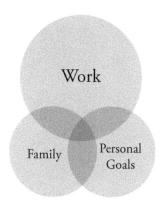

FIGURE I.2 A LIFE OUT OF PROPORTION

The ultimate danger is when this state devolves into complete disparity. When our lives fracture in this way (Figure 1.3), it manifests as "dis-ease" of the body, mind, and spirit: pain, illness, discomfort; anxiety, stress, depression; listlessness, apathy, disassociation; fatigue, exhaustion, lack of will. And these issues may contribute to, or even become, clinical illnesses: high blood pressure, arthritis, fibromyalgia, chronic fatigue, mental health disorders, endocrine imbalance, cancer, and more. In Traditional Chinese Medicine the imbalance of one aspect of the self—whether it be body (Jing), spirit (Shen), or energy (Qi)—affects the entire self. In other words, mental states create physical illness, and physical illness creates mental states. The more fractured our day-to-day existence seems to us, the more our serenity and joy are replaced by anxiety and exasperation, which is fertile ground for illness.

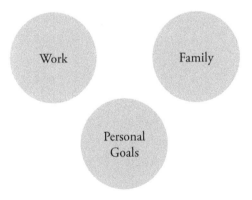

FIGURE 1.3 A DISJUNCT LIFE

This state of "dis-ease" can have positive ramifications, though. As Chuang-Tzu remarks, "Society seeks when there is chaos" (Cleary 1992, p.66). Illness and imbalance can be the necessary catalysts for people to reestablish harmony, balance, and value. Many people who have the initial desire to study meditation, Qigong, Taiji, or to learn about Buddhism or Taoism with me, for example, chronicle their stories of their struggles with physical or mental health issues, stress, anxiety, a chronic condition, or they are coping with being the caregiver for an ailing spouse, partner, parent, or loved one. The problems that people face in their lives may incite them to actively seek better health and well-being.

Dual Cultivation: Awareness and Energy

The identification of stress, illness, and imbalance is a vital first step to initiating a return to balance, but it also opens up the even more difficult matter of *how*: How do we reintegrate our lives? How do we find the means and the tools to live a life of balance? How do we get to the other side of the tunnel where there is a beautiful vista and a flowing river? This is the basic question of this book. The two most significant and fundamental qualities that need to be cultivated are awareness and energy. The initial recognition of disharmony begins the process of defining the nature of the problem and marks the need for a course of action. The awakening of awareness must look back to perceive the elements that brought the person to this particular difficulty as well as a forward glance to a path that leads out of it. The character and historical context of the problem and the necessity for action—the what and how—come into clearer focus, which sparks the understanding regarding the energy needed to fully address the issue.

Awareness shares a dynamic relationship with energy, with each complementing the other. The Taiji classics state that "Yi leads Qi" (intentional mind leads energy). Awareness directs the energy toward a specific goal. Energy is required both to sustain the individual's awareness as well as to continue on the path toward wholeness. Awareness and energy are two interrelated things that need to be cultivated simultaneously in order to work together to reach well-being, health, and balance. This relationship might best be represented as a simple equation (Figure 1.4).

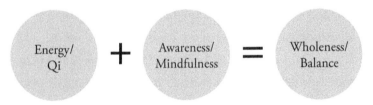

FIGURE I.4 ENERGY EQUATION

The heart of the matter is how to maintain awareness as well as generate the energy required to sustain that awareness. When the two are disintegrated, awareness wanes. When a person is tired, for example, any careless action (tripping, causing an accident, and the like) is directly related to not having the energy to focus; or when we are worn out, we cannot muster the concentration required for a particularly difficult task. Quite simply, mindful attention requires sustained energy. Energy and awareness play off one another in a dance that fuels focus, direction, and drive. Taoism represents this relationship as the universal principle of the Tao and the perpetual transforming of Yin and Yang (Figure 1.5).

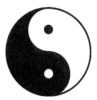

FIGURE 1.5 YIN/YANG SYMBOL

Yang is present within Yin (represented as the circle of black within the white), and Yin is present within Yang (the white circle within the black). Each is in the perpetual process of becoming the other. As Yang reaches its apex, Yin has already begun, and vice versa. The ongoing process corrects, balances, and perpetuates itself without interference.

If the terms of Yin and Yang are translated as awareness and energy, the same principles hold true. Energy fuels awareness, and awareness fuels energy. Consciousness without energy is the state of recognizing the problem of imbalance in life, but not having the means to rectify and address the situation; energy without awareness is to have unfocused energy without purpose.

Since awareness and energy share a dynamic relationship, it is important to understand the energy that fuels living—specifically, where it comes from, how we use it, and how we can cultivate it. In Chinese philosophy, this energy, which is called Qi (also spelled Chi or Ki), flows from a number of sources. We are born with Qi (called Yuan Qi or prenatal energy, which we get from our mothers), and we receive energy from various outside sources such as the food that we eat, our environments, and from rest. The Chinese ideogram for Qi (Figure 1.6) points directly to the most essential ingredients for our survival: food and air.

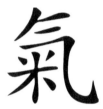

FIGURE 1.6 CHINESE CHARACTER FOR QI

The ideogram itself is composed of the signs for air (top and to the right) and uncooked rice (bottom left). To translate this ideogram into a more contemporary model requires merely looking at the basic scientific rendering of energy: Energy is Input minus Output ($E = I - O$). Human energy, though, extends beyond mere food and air, and includes the mental, emotional, and psychological elements as well. For example, a partial list includes some of the necessities required to maintain the physical body alongside things that sustain us as social creatures as well (Table 1.1).

TABLE 1.1 INPUT AND OUTPUT OF ENERGY

INPUT (POSITIVE)	OUTPUT (NEGATIVE)
Healthy food	Processed food/empty calories
Rest/sleep	Poor, inadequate sleep
Energy-boosting exercise	Energy-depleting exercise
Healthy environments	Polluted, toxic environments
Positive emotions	Negative emotions
Calm mental states	Anxiety, stress
Healthy, supportive relationships	Negative, stressful relationships
Purposeful work	Meaningless tasks

An item can and often does cross into both the positive and negative categories. All food, for example, requires energy to digest and convert it into useable nutrients, but some food is made up of empty calories that do not contribute to overall well-being. The choice between an apple and candy is a clear example of such a qualitative act that impacts the body and its energy. The differentiation is qualitative choices between an output that exceeds its input or one where the input exceeds the output. A choice can deplete or replenish.

The energy potential should be weighed carefully with each choice. Those choices can be shaped by emotional and psychological dynamics, and mindfulness is not merely focused upon the external but the internal as well. In other words, sometimes a "meaningless task" becomes purposeful work. For example, when irritated or annoyed, washing the dishes may seem like a waste of valuable time and energy, but when a person is in a good mood, that household chore may be a positive reminder of the enjoyable time entertaining and eating. Our internal psychological landscape filters how we perceive the world, but in the matter of energy, that internal state (such as anger, anxiety, sadness, and other emotions) contributes to the depletion or the cultivation of energy. Such consciousness constantly observes and monitors how energy is being used.

Given this principle of the relationship between input and output, as well as the inextricable quality of awareness and energy, the ultimate goal is to maximize inputs and minimize outputs, thereby increasing the level of energy; or as Grandmaster Wu often says, "Save more, spend less." The accepted contemporary standard, though, seems more akin to a rechargeable battery on so many of our electronic devices. If we translate the battery into human terms, we wake up with a certain amount of energy (say 100% capacity), and each task throughout the day drains the battery until it is low. At that point, we rest and recharge. Unfortunately, like those batteries, our maximum capacity seems to diminish as we age, leading to more and more fatigue, stress, and restlessness. Unlike our electronic devices, we cannot "upgrade" our bodies.

Fortunately, our bodies aren't merely batteries, and when working with meditation, Taiji, Qigong, and other Internal Arts that focus on the vitality of Qi, it is possible to increase our energetic capacity and return to a more efficient physical, emotional, and psychological state. In fact, the result of many of these practices is an increase to the maximum level of daily energy. For example, if the basic energy unit per day is ten, over time that gradually increases to eleven, then fifteen, and so forth. The goal is to accumulate more energy at the end of the day than the end of the previous day. The process is one of cultivation and growth.

We might compare the generation and retention of energy to weather-proofing our homes. When we make our homes more energy efficient, we take steps to make sure that windows and doors are properly sealed, there are adequate levels of insulation throughout the walls and ceilings, and monitor that the furnace is working at an efficient level, thereby minimizing the loss of heat. If we increase the level of input and reduce the level of outputs by installing a more fuel-efficient, high-capacity furnace as well as better windows and doors, then we reduce the loss of energy even more. Weather-proofing is based upon the principle of anti-depletion, and with the retention of heat (which along with light is energy or Qi) there is the added benefit of cost-cutting. Energy (fuel) is still required to heat the house, but the amount of fuel required to sustain a certain temperature as well as the amount of energy lost is reduced.

The same principle applies to our own energy, and the list of inputs and outputs includes not only physical but also emotional and psychological processes by which energy is generated as well as depleted. In the same way that we analyze the fuel efficiency of a house for weather-proofing, we need to carefully examine three different but interrelated aspects of ourselves: our physical body as well as our psychological and emotional processes, which are Yi (wisdom mind) and Xin (emotional mind). To cultivate Qi is to look inward and outward—at the processes by which external energy is absorbed and the internal response that uses, stores, or disperses that energy. Lao Tzu's words from the *Tao Te Ching* are extremely poignant in respect to the process behind "Qi efficiency":

> *Those who know others are wise;*
> *Those who know themselves are enlightened.*
> *Those who overcome others are powerful;*
> *Those who overcome themselves are strong.*
>
> (CLEARY 1992, P.29)

Our awareness is like a pane of glass through which we observe the external world, but that view also turns inward illuminating our responses to that stimuli. Our awareness illuminates ourselves, our world, and our path. The purpose is nothing less than self-knowledge and mastery.

The recognition of life imbalance is the initial spark for investigating the nature of the problem as well as a search for resolution. Our motivation awakens a force for change that becomes the Will of Qi, which has a number of qualities: discipline, drive, focus, perseverance, resolve, desire. The initial intentional charge sets the entire process in motion: the will to change, the will to be aware, the will to cultivate Qi. We embark upon a path to become healthier, happier, more balanced, and more at harmony with the world. As we continue on that path, we gain focus, deepen our awareness, and our vitality and energy noticeably increase. As we feel healthier and more balanced, this validates the process, thereby providing the reinforcement to continue on the path of developing oneself in this manner. The danger, though, is falling into complacency (what Thoreau calls "resignation") thereby losing the drive to continue on the path, and sometimes the greatest obstacle is satisfaction. When we feel good, healthy, and whole, we are less motivated to continue investing in the choices and actions that brought us back to health. Simply put, people lose motivation when they think things are fixed—ignoring what it was that they have been doing that brought about their current state of peace, wholeness, and harmony. By shirking the very practices that healed them, they return to a fractured sense of self.

While discipline and drive cannot be passively transferred from one person to another, what *can* be taught are the tools to develop body and mind practices that enhance awareness and energy and thereby fuel Will by reintegrating the self and generating a more harmonious relationship with the world. Intention illuminates awareness and awakens the energy to sustain and continue. While Will sparks the process of awakening, Qi is the driving force that reintegrates and unites. Awareness is fueled by Qi and drives our Will. At the very heart of this ongoing process, Qi is the force of life that sustains our body as well as our mind and spirit.

Qi can be transformative when it is applied to our mindful watching and realigning of the internal and external landscapes that constitute ourselves and our worlds. We should keep in mind the rally call of the German poet Rainer Maria Rilke, who concludes his poem "The Archaic Torso of Apollo" with the stern urging: "You must change your life" (Mitchell 1989, p.61). To change from a fractured disintegrated self (just a torso) to one of wholeness (a complete body) requires the courage to look closely at the patterns, habits, and perceptions of oneself and the world. And it requires continuous energy to stay the course, which is not a one-step process or one that is ever completed. It is an ever evolving path of looking, revising, focusing, discovering, and pursuing. To have the resolve to continue discovering the depths of purpose and value requires a continuous influx of Qi, and it requires the courage to remain on the never-ending journey toward wholeness and completion of the body, breath, mind, Qi, and spirit.

Living Qi

Everything we do has an underlying purpose: when we wash the dishes, we are cleaning these things to be used again; when we get in our cars, we are traveling to a certain destination—or if we are on a leisurely drive, we are relaxing and taking in the scenery; when we sit down to read a book, we are taking some quiet time for learning about a subject of interest. The same holds true with the practices of mediation, Taiji, Qigong, and other Internal Arts. An underlying purpose is there: to become healthier, happier, a better person. The more deeply we look, we discover that our actions and thoughts extend beyond the surface as well. The classics state "练拳不练功, 到老一场空," which translates as "Even if you practice your whole life, if you practice form but not gong, your art will be empty." The quote is specifically addressing Taiji, but it equally applies to living in general. "Gong" has both a physical and a mental meaning. To practice "gong" means to work on physical balance, coordination of movement, ability, flexibility, sensitivity, and strength. It also means the cultivation of awareness, confidence, and the tranquility of heart and mind.

To incorporate the essence of "gong" into life is to move beyond the superficial and into a deeper, more satisfying relationship with oneself and the world. It was Henry David Thoreau who remarked that his purpose behind retreating to the woods at Walden Pond was to truly engage in the act of living:

I went to the woods because I wished to live deliberately, to front only the essential facts of life, and see if I could not learn what it had to teach, and not, when I came to die, discover that I had not lived. I did not wish to live what was not life, living is so dear; nor did I wish to practice resignation, unless it was quite necessary. I wanted to live deep and suck out all the marrow of life, to live so sturdily and Spartan-like as to put to rout all that was not life, to cut a broad swath and shave close, to drive life into a corner, and reduce it to its lowest terms, and, if it proved to be mean, why then to get the whole and genuine meanness of it, and publish its meanness to the world; or if it were sublime, to know it by experience, and be able to give a true account of it in my next excursion. (Sayre 1985, pp.394–395)

If we look at the Taoist lesson behind Lie Yukou's "The Man Who Wanted to Forget," his madness is the only escape he can imagine from the mundane quality of his life. Incapable of discerning the essential from the nonessential, his only joy and serenity comes when he has a complete break with reality. "Gong" is not escape, but the immersion into the real, which awakens the tranquility of heart and mind. Living deeply requires looking deeply and honestly to discover the profound yet simple reality beneath the surface.

One of my Taiji students, who has studied with me for over ten years but has been a student of other marital arts for forty-plus years, once remarked that focusing upon "gong" made a remarkable transformation to his practice and his life. He explained to me, "I realized that for all of those years of training I had been skirting the internal work. And when I began to do that work, it was as if I realized I had been taking a shower with a raincoat on"; or to put it a different way, my student had discovered the meaning behind the classic saying "Hua Quan Xiu Tui," which literally means "flower fist, brocade leg" but refers to something that is beautiful but useless. His training up to that point was useless, but once he began training in a purposeful way, the transformation was readily apparent to him and to others: he was able to relax, sleep better, feel his Qi, root his body, let go of his anger, and enjoy life. To revise your art and your life—and to maintain that trajectory along that path—requires tremendous hard work for the student as well as the teacher, who must distill, model, and be the essence of "gong fu"—hard, disciplined work.

From a teaching standpoint, it certainly is easier to explain the surface than to attempt to plumb the depths of a subject since the teacher not only has to be an expert on the subject but also a paradigm of behavior with the necessary tools to convey that expertise to others. The word for such tools in Sanskrit is *upaya* or skillful means. To try to show how to improve living is a Herculean task, and while it is much easier to teach the choreography of the forms—and from the side of the student, to be a form collector rather than an internal martial artist—I wanted to tackle this task by imparting some of the essential techniques that move beyond the surface, penetrate into the depths of practices, and drive toward the heart of Qi. This book builds upon my twenty-plus years as a Taiji player, student, and teacher, as well as my training as Ch'an (Zen) monk and priest, and the many years I spent as a university professor, father, husband, healer, scholar, and human being. If I had to reduce the goal of my book down to one maxim, it would be the classic saying "The most important thing in learning martial arts is to practice in the proper way." The proper path of practicing and living encompasses all facets of "gong"—the physical, mental, and spiritual. During my time as a teacher of the Internal Arts, philosophy, Taoism, Buddhism, and life, I have distilled the essence of some of these seemingly disparate areas into a range of tools to generate purpose and value for individual practice and to create harmony, balance, and wholeness.

This book takes place at the intersection of practice and theory, providing a unique perspective of the roles of body, breath, and mind for Qi, the vital life energy, as well as the rich philosophical tradition and history of that energy. The book delves deeply into Traditional Chinese Medicine, Taoism, Buddhism, the Internal Martial Arts, Qigong, and the philosophy and history of Qi in order to present a fresh perspective of the hows and whys of Qi: how it is created, how it has been used, and how it can be refined for health, healing, well-being, and spiritual work. While other books concentrate upon either theory or practice— either as studies of the philosophy of Taoism, Buddhism, Traditional Chinese Medicine or as training manuals on specific techniques or styles—this book bridges theory and practice to show how to generate Qi, why the regulation of Qi is important, and how that relates to these various philosophical and spiritual traditions.

CHAPTER 2

Returning to the Source
The History of Energy and Its Uses

Energy surged through the conference room. Nearly one hundred people were pouncing and clawing like tigers, prancing like deer, staggering like upright bears, plucking peaches from tree branches like monkeys, and soaring like cranes. Dr. Jwing-Ming Yang was poised at the front of the room leading everyone through the Five Animals Sport Qigong (Wu Qin Xi), the famous set attributed to Huatuo, a Chinese Medicine doctor from the second century CE who is often credited with finalizing the first "therapeutic" Qigong set that harmonizes the five Yin organs of the body in order to maintain health. During a much needed break, someone asked Dr. Yang why Western culture lagged so far behind when it came to Qi, and without missing a beat, he replied, "Because all of the people who worked with energy and who were attuned to the natural world in early Europe were burned as witches." The historical continuity of energy work in the West was broken when the people who knew it and could teach it were silenced, and the gap created has been difficult to overcome. Dr. Yang's historical insight about the implications of the witch hunts not only struck me as extremely profound, but it also emphasized that the concept of energy or Qi is not the sole property of ancient Chinese thought. In fact, similar words and concepts can be found throughout a wide range of culture and history. A partial listing of such ideas from a number of cultures include: *Prana* in Hindu; *Ki* in Japanese; *Pneuma* in Ancient Greek; *Lüng* in Tibetan; *Mana* in Hawaiian; *Ruah* in Hebrew; *Bioelectricity* in contemporary scientific language; and even *The Force* in the pop cultural language of the *Star Wars* movies. Many of these concepts from around the world emphasize certain qualities such as breath, power, spirit, process, evolution, intention, and more—suggesting that Qi's reach extends beyond cultural boundaries and historical periods.

While Chinese philosophy does not own the idea of Qi or vital energy, its history and philosophy offers the most detailed analysis. Within Chinese thought and practice, Qi is the foundational cornerstone of Traditional Chinese Medicine, Taoist and Buddhist philosophy, Martial Arts training, and more. But Qi extends beyond abstract ideas and philosophical discussion. Within that worldview, everything is the product and the sign of Qi. It is the architectural material *and* the process by which the physical world comes into being—including the human body. To properly cultivate Qi requires an understanding of its history—how it is perceived as operating in the world, its principles, and how it functions. As the contemporary Taoist master Deng Ming-Dao asks in his *Everyday Tao* (1996), "Isn't it better to stand on the shoulders of the previous generation? ... Rather than invent everything, it might be better if we first learned to do things the classic way" (p.40). The process of learning the classic way is not meant to be an academic exercise, but one that tests, refines, and uses. And to study what has come before isn't blind acceptance of those ways as sacred, but rather a learning process that applies and adapts. In this spirit of learning, this chapter explores how Qi has been, and continues to be, the key to health, healing, and well-being as well as spiritual cultivation, and having a deeper understanding of its history reveals how it can be used to enhance the act of living.

The Qi of Health

The principle of Qi can be found in many historical sources—from the *I Ching* (also known as *Book of Changes*) to Martial Arts and meditation manuals—but more so than any other source, *The Yellow Emperor's Guide to Internal Medicine*, or *Huangti Neijing*, offers the most profound insights into the life of Qi. *The Yellow Emperor's Guide to Internal Medicine* shapes the core of Chinese culture, thought, and worldview, and all other aspects of that culture, whether they be Confucian, Buddhist, Taoist, or something else, are branches that grow from its roots. The book is attributed to Huang Ti, the Yellow Emperor, who ruled from 2697 to 2597 BCE and is credited with initiating Chinese culture. The date of the composition of the book may be uncertain (many scholars place it around 1000 BCE) and its authorship by Huang Ti would not hold true since his rule was over 1500 years earlier, but its place as the most significant text in Chinese Medicine theory is certain, and the discussions and theories within its pages brilliantly illuminate the nature of Qi and its functions within the larger world as well as the human body.

The structure of *The Yellow Emperor's Guide to Internal Medicine* is a dialogue between Huang Ti and Qi Bo, one of the Emperor's ministers, and those conversations outline the principle of the Way (or Tao) of the universe and how its identifiable processes apply to internal medicine, diseases, and the treatment of those diseases. The central premise of the book is that the Tao and health are deeply interconnected. When Huang Ti asked for an elaboration upon that connection, Qi Bo replied:

In the past, people practiced the Tao, the Way of Life. They understood the principle of balance, of yin and yang, as represented by the transformation of the energies of the universe. Thus, they formulated practices such as Dao-yin, an exercise combining stretching, massaging, and breathing to promote energy flow, and meditation to help maintain and harmonize themselves with the universe. They ate a balanced diet at regular times, arose and retired at regular hours, avoided overstressing their bodies and minds, and refrained from overindulgence of all kinds. They maintained well-being of body and mind; thus, it is not surprising that they lived over one hundred years.

These days, people have changed their way of life. They drink wine as though it were water, indulge excessively in destructive activities, drain their jing—the body's essence that is stored in the kidneys—and deplete their qi. They do not know the secret of conserving their energy and vitality. Seeking emotional excitement and momentary pleasures, people disregard the natural rhythm and order of the universe. They fail to regulate their lifestyle and diet, and sleep improperly. So it is not surprising that they look old at fifty and die soon after. (Ni 1995, p.1)

This basic conception of health and energy is so fundamental that over 1000 years later *Wen tzu*, one of the great Taoist sourcebooks which is also known by the title *Understanding the Mysteries*, reiterates these same ideas:

The way of developed people is to cultivate the body by calmness and nurture life by frugality...to govern the body and nurture essence, sleep and rest moderately, eat and drink appropriately; harmonize emotions, simplify activities. Those who are inwardly attentive to the self attain this and are immune to pervasive energies. (Cleary 2003a, p.147)

The primary focus of *The Yellow Emperor's Guide to Internal Medicine* is medical—although, as evident from the quote from *Wen tzu*, it touches upon many concepts and traditions that extend well beyond disease and healing. Nevertheless, the discussions of Qi Bo and Huang Ti elaborate upon Qi and how an understanding of Qi can be used by Traditional Chinese Medicine in diagnosis, analysis, and treatment. To better understand just how pervasive and profound these ideas are, it is necessary to provide a sketch of some basic principles of Traditional Chinese Medicine and especially how those ideas relate to Qi. The centrality of Qi and its role for health and healing will be clearer when placed within the context of these fundamental principles.

The Qi of Traditional Chinese Medicine

The human body is composed of three things: Qi, Jing, and Shen. Vital energy, or Qi, functions alongside Jing (usually translated as "essence" that is stored in the kidneys and is inherited from both parents) and Shen (usually translated as "spirit" but is more akin to awareness and consciousness), which Qi Bo exclaims "rules all mental and creative function." Jing is part of the body's instinctual organic process, while Shen is conscious action. A person's Jing is established at birth, while Shen can be cultivated through various practices. Like Shen, Qi can be increased and refined as well. One ancient Taoist source titled *Vitality, Energy, Spirit* states quite simply, "The human body is only vitality, energy, and spirit. Vitality, energy, and spirit are called the three treasures" (Cleary 1991a, p.73). Qi, Jing,

Shen—vitality, energy, spirit—constitute the human body as a whole and each are central to health and overall well-being. But Qi is the force operating within Jing and Shen.

Everything in the universe has Qi, but the human body is composed of two main types: *prenatal Qi*, which we inherit through our parents and in more scientific language is a part of our genetic mapping and DNA; and *postnatal Qi*, which includes grain Qi (derived from what we eat) and air Qi (from the air that we breathe and from the environment). As stated in Chapter 1, the Chinese character for Qi is made up of these two images—one for uncooked rice (grain Qi) and the other for air (air Qi)—which, when combined, form postnatal Qi.

These two major types of Qi are also broken down into even more detailed categories that correspond to specific functions and processes within the body:

- *Organ Qi (Zang fu zhi qi).* Each organ in the body has its own quality of Qi.

- *Nutritive Qi (Ying qi).* Associated with the circulatory system, this is the Qi that feeds the body and is represented by the saying that "Qi is the force behind the blood."

- *Meridian Qi (Jing luo zhi qi).* This Qi flows through the channels and pathways of the body and connects the organs and limbs.

- *Protective Qi (Wei qi).* This Qi protects the body from external influences such as bacteria, viruses, and other environmental factors that can infect and sicken the body.

- *Ancestral Qi or the Qi of the chest (Zong qi).* This Qi governs and facilitates respiration and heart function.

In *The Yellow Emperor's Guide to Internal Medicine*, Huang Ti and Qi Bo also discuss a number of different functions and purposes of Qi within the body.

- Qi is the source of movement both in terms of physical muscular motion, the involuntary movement of the heart and lungs, intentional action and thinking, and the human life cycle of birth, growth, and aging.

- Qi protects the body by negating what are called "pernicious external influences" (e.g., bacteria, viruses, environmental toxins) that once they invade the body can manifest as illness or disease.

- Qi transforms nutrients into the fluids of the body such as blood, tears, sweat, and urine. Qi is the agent that balances and harmonizes the intake and processing of food and the elimination of waste products.

- Qi is the governing force for the organs of the body and "holds" the organs in place as well as preventing the excessive loss of bodily fluids.

- Qi warms the body by maintaining and regulating the temperature of the organs, limbs, and extremities.

Qi is not inactive and stationary, but flows through various channels, paths, and meridians in order to maintain and regulate the body as a whole. Balance and health depend on the pathways through the body being open, the Qi not being obstructed, excessive, or deficient, and there being smooth and unimpeded communication between all of the organs, muscles, tendons, and the skeletal, nervous, and lymphatic systems.

Essentially, according to Chinese Medicine, twelve primary channels or meridians pass through the body and are related to the Lung, Large Intestine, Stomach, Spleen, Heart, Small Intestine, Bladder, Kidney, Pericardium, Triple Burner, Gall Bladder, and Liver. These channels form a loop throughout the body, and the second section of *The Yellow Emperor's Guide to Internal Medicine* focuses upon these pathways since any blockage, deficiency, or excess in these pathways creates illness. These pathways are used in acupuncture treatments as a way to reharmonize and balance the Qi of the body. In addition to the twelve meridian channels, Qi also flows through the eight extraordinary vessels. These vessels are named the Governing Channel (up the back of the torso), the Conception Channel (down the front of the torso), the Thrusting Channel (on the inside of the spinal column connecting the top of the head [Baihui] with the base of the spine [Huiyin]), the Girdle Vessel (around the waist), the Yin (inside and upward flowing) and Yang (outside downward flowing) channels of the legs, and the Yin (inside and upward flowing) and Yang (outside and downward flowing) channels of the arms. The twelve primary meridians and the eight extraordinary channels are the major Qi causeways of the body.[1] When those pathways are open, and the Qi is balanced and smooth, the individual is healthy.

Qi can be further defined as having either a Yin or a Yang aspect. Yang and Yin are usually translated as the Bright Side of the Hill (Yang) and the Dark Side of the Hill (Yin), and stand in contrast to one another. For example, Yang is male, day, light, sun, destruction, and action; Yin is female, night, moon, productive, and still. The relationship between the two is rendered as a swirling ball of Yin and Yang that is engaged in an infinite dance of harmonizing, balancing, generating, and destroying. The rising and falling of Yin and Yang generates the material forms of the universe, which are called the "ten thousand things," and so the observable physical world is in fact one moment in the process of Yin and Yang energy coming into and out of being. Huang Ti states this most directly: "The law of yin and yang is the natural order of the universe, the foundation of all things, mother of all changes, the root of life and death" (Ni 1995, p.47). The flow of Qi, as embodied by the play of Yin and Yang, is the general and the specific rule of the universe, and the signature of the Tao.

This flow of energy permeates everything in an ever swirling circle, which is the heart of the universe. Not surprisingly this concept of Qi is the centerpiece of the ancient Chinese story of the creation of space and time too. That story proposes that in the beginning was a void and boundless state called Wuji, which means "no polarity." A force called *Taiji* (which is not to be confused with the Internal Art, Taiji) splits Wuji into two poles—Yin and Yang—and from Yin and Yang all things come into being. Lao Tzu recounts this story in Chapter 42 of *Tao Te Ching*:

> *The Way produces one;*
> *One produces two,*
> *Two produce three,*
> *Three produce all beings;*
> *All beings bear yin and embrace yang,*
> *With a mellowing energy for harmony.*
>
> (CLEARY 1992, P.35)

The story of Wuji (the one) being split into two emphasizes the role of Yin and Yang within all beings, and the natural process is one of harmonizing energy. Such "mellowing energy" for Huang Ti is the sign of health and well-being.

Since Yin and Yang together form a "universal" concept, that universality is extended to the body, which is composed of Yin and Yang organs that are connected through the channels and meridians. The Yin organs (called "Zang" organs by Huang Ti) are Liver, Heart, Spleen, Lung, and Kidney, and their main quality is that they "store and do not drain," which means that their function is to create homeostasis (balance) within the body. The Yang organs (called "Fu") include the Gall Bladder, Small Intestine, Large Intestine, Stomach, Bladder, and Triple Burner, and these organs "drain and do not store," which means that their function is to process and move food and waste products. The balance and sustenance of the organs depend on the pathways through the body being open and thereby allowing for a smooth communication of Qi between all of the organs, muscles, tendons, and the skeletal, nervous, and lymph systems.

Yin and Yang are the two poles—or extremes—of all the energy of the universe, but Qi is not merely one or the other but is engaged in an ongoing process like a wave cresting, crashing, retreating, and reformulating. The interplay of Yin and Yang is recast and refined through another of Huang Ti's theories—the Five Elements Theory, wherein the elements of Wood, Fire, Earth, Metal, and Water are intermediaries within the poles of Yin and Yang (Figure 2.1). The Five Elements are energetic processes that take on material form in the same way that Yin and Yang combined construct a "thing," and while an object may be predominately one element, it is interdependent upon all of the others. A piece of physical wood is Wood element, for example, but it is also made up of all of the other elements—most easily recognized in Water and Earth (nutrients)—all of which combine in a process that manifests as a material moment or form. The Five Elements Theory is another perspective of the energetic Yin/Yang processes of the natural world through their relationships, which are both constructive (Yin) and destructive (Yang), rather than a way to categorize material objects. The energetic constructive process of the elements is that Wood creates Fire; Fire creates Earth; Earth creates Metal; Metal creates

Water; and Water creates Wood. There is also a destructive energetic sequence as well: Wood weakens Earth; Earth limits Water; Fire conquers Metal; Metal cuts Wood; and Water extinguishes Fire.

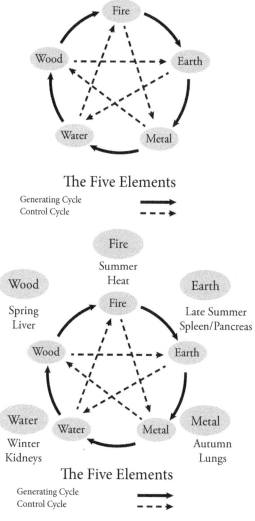

FIGURE 2.1A AND B FIVE ELEMENTS THEORY

These elements also correspond to the seasons: Wood = spring; Fire = summer; Earth = late summer; Metal = autumn; and Water = winter. The seasonal cycle of the year illustrates the process of this energetic cycle and how that cycle is observable in the physical world. If the elemental process was put into a story of the energy of the seasons, it might read: As the ice of winter begins to melt (Yin dissipating as Yang begins to rise), the water awakens the trees and plants, which sparks spring growth (Yang awakens) that explodes into full fiery summer bloom (high Yang). As autumn approaches (Yang begins to dissipate), trees begin to drop leaves like metal cutting wood in order to conserve energy and water for the approach of winter (high Yin).

Such a cycle corresponds to a human life as well. We are born, grow, flourish, decline, wither, and die. *Taoist Meditations: Methods for Cultivating a Healthy Mind and Body* states the relationship in simple terms: "Nature has five forces—metal, wood, water, fire, and earth... These five forces are inherent in the human body, where they constitute the five organs—heart, liver, pancreas, lungs, and kidneys": Wood = Liver; Fire = Heart; Earth = Spleen/Pancreas; Metal = Lung; and Water = Kidney (Cleary 2000, p.13). The health of the body depends on a systematic balance of the organs and their processes— and especially between the Yin and Yang organs and the channels and meridians that feed those organs. Such a state of balance within the body is the state of supreme health.

The way of health depends on the flowing and quality of Qi within the human body.

Qi from Theory to Practice

The reach and influence of *The Yellow Emperor's Guide to Internal Medicine* extends beyond the use of Qi to enhance health and maintain life, but at its core, the detailed analysis of Qi and how it can be used focuses on the medical diagnoses, treatments, and healing modalities. According to Livia Kohn in her *Chinese Healing Exercises* (2008), "Health and long life come through working with *qi* to the best of one's ability, attaining a state of perfect balance, utmost harmony, and complete self-fulfillment" (p.3). The discussions include a range of modalities such as herbs, acupuncture, Daoyin, Qigong, and meditation—all of which are mentioned throughout *The Yellow Emperor's Guide to Internal Medicine* as means of regulating Qi and sustaining health. But the practices of Daoyin, Qigong, and meditation play extremely significant roles in Taoist and Buddhist practices.

Qi Bo refers to the value of Qigong when he praises sages who use exercises that combine "stretching, massaging, and breathing to promote energy flow" as well as the healers who use these "practices and methods...to contact pathogens without becoming ill" (Ni 1995, pp.22, 414). Qigong, which literally translates as energy (Qi) work (gong), are sets of exercises that couple movement with deep breathing and focused mental concentration.

Authentic Qigong sets, such as Five Animals, Eight Pieces of Brocade, and others, draw upon the theories of Qi, Yin and Yang organs, channels, and meridians, and the Five Elements Theory as espoused by Huang Ti and Qi Bo—and such Qigong utilizes and advances these principles in order to form an extremely effective tool for correcting and maintaining physical and mental health and well-being.

The Five Animals Sport (Wu Qin Xi) is widely regarded as one of the earliest therapeutic Qigong sets. Attributed to Huatou, who either invented or refined the set into its final version during the second century CE, the form builds upon the movements of the Tiger, Deer, Bear, Monkey, and Crane. Each of those animals, in turn, is linked to a Yin organ: Tiger/Liver; Deer/Kidney; Bear/Spleen; Monkey/Heart; and Crane/Lung. Each animal within the set has a number of specific movements that bend, stretch, and massage the channels and organs. By extending, circling, and undulating the body, the Qi is stimulated through the organs and their channels, and the diaphragmatic breathing is used to massage the organ by applying and releasing pressure. The overarching purpose is to stimulate the Qi to flow evenly through the channels, thereby correcting any blockages or deficiences, and sustaining the body's overall health.

Qigong is often conceptualized as a modality for health and healing that builds upon the Yellow Emperor's theories. As *Practical Taoism*, a Taoist sourcebook, states, "Energy is life increasing medicine" (Cleary 1996, p.32). And while Taoist practice asserts that "the quintessence of the science of essence and life is to gather primal energy," that use of energy extends beyond health and healing and is used for spiritual cultivation in both Taoism and Buddhism. While Chinese Buddhism is best known for meditation and Shaolin-style Kung Fu rather than its Qigong and the emphasis on internal energy work, Ch'an Buddhism has a rich history of Qigong. An exploration of how Qi fits into that history reveals a great deal about how the use of Qi extends beyond health and healing and into the realm of meditation and the cultivation of spiritual awareness.

The Qi of Waking Up

Qigong plays an important role in the history of Ch'an (Zen in Japanese) Buddhism in China. Bodhidharma, the first patriarch of Ch'an Buddhism, is credited with initiating Ch'an with its blending of Indian (Theravadan) Buddhism with Taoism and Chinese culture. Bodhidharma was an Indian prince who traveled to China in the fifth or sixth century CE, and after fleeing from a meeting with Emperor Wu (Xiao Yan), who he may have offended, Bodhidharma sought shelter at the Shaolin Temple. When he arrived he was disturbed to find the monks at the temple in poor physical condition. Supposedly he retreated to a cave to meditate for seven or nine years depending on the version of the story. Some versions of the story claim that Bodhidharma was refused entry to the temple, and so he retreated to the cave until he was allowed inside. Nevertheless, when he emerged from the cave to teach, he had formulated a number of training methods—most notably Eighteen Arhat Hands, Shi Ba Lo Han Gong, which heavily influenced the Shaolin style of Kung Fu, and a number of Qigong sets including the famous Muscle and Tendon Changing Classic, Yi Jin Jing, as well as Bone and Marrow Washing, Xi Sui Jing. Scholars disagree whether Bodhidharma created these forms, synthesized them from other styles, or was given credit to these forms that were developed hundreds of years later. Whether Bodhidharma created these forms or not is secondary to this discussion of Qi, though, since what is relevant is that the Ch'an tradition incorporated and continues to emphasize these Qi-based exercises as part of its authentic lineage and practice. The important question is not did he create these forms, but rather how is Qi central to Ch'an practices? The answer reveals much about how Qi can be used to increase the quality of life beyond physical health.

While the Shaolin Temple is famous for its Kung Fu, Bodhidharma's inclusion of Qigong forms emphasizes the important role that Qi plays with Ch'an. The poor physical condition of the monks was a major hindrance for the central aspect of Ch'an's emphasis upon meditation, which requires an abundance of strength, stamina, and energy. In one of Bodhidharma's teachings called "The Breakthrough Sutra" he explains that "the most essential method, which includes all other methods, is beholding the mind" (Pine 1987, p.77). Concentrated awareness is meant to be sustained while sitting, moving, doing chores, and all other moments of conscious activity. To be able to continuously behold the mind is fully waking up and becoming an enlightened being.

This meditative approach requires sustained concentration, awareness, and stamina, and poor physical condition would be a major detriment for the success of the individual practitioner. When Bodhidharma encountered the monks and regarded them as lacking strength and stamina, it was both an internal and external weakness, and his response was to formulate and teach two different methods that emphasized training the physical body and its internal landscape. Both training techniques cultivate, gather, and strengthen Qi, and while that person would gain greater health, the explicit purpose is to use that Qi for awareness. In the language of the Three Treasures of Qi, Jing, and Shen, the Qi is cultivated to feed Shen. In turn, Shen is used to "see" the world as it is. The individual would pierce through the veil of personal subjectivity and the relative perspective of the ego that obscures the world as it is. The basic premise of Buddhist philosophy as a whole, regardless of its particular school, is that our egos (constructed selves) obscure and filter reality into a limited or even false view that perpetuates the state of suffering that Buddhism proposes marks all human existence. To "wake up" is to recognize this subjectivity and to see the world "as it is." Such waking up in Ch'an marks the liberation from suffering.

Such an awareness enables the person to interact with the world more appropriately. The original character for Ch'an is a transliteration of the Sanskrit word *dhyana*, which means "meditative absorption." (Similarly, Ch'an was transcribed as "Zen" in Japanese.) The Chinese conception of such absorption was an intimacy with oneself (called one's inherent Buddha nature) and the world, both of which are inseparable from each other. Learning how to best interact with the world is called *upayana* in Sanskrit, which means "skillful means," and is the tool of addressing the world. This meditative tool is about being able to see the patterns of Qi that characterize a situation, and in seeing these patterns, recognizing that the situation may require a more delicate "Yin" response or a thunderous contribution of "Yang" in order to transform a situation into one of waking up and liberation. Such a technique is akin to the skillful use of an oar to steer across the river. The river (the flow of Qi that creates human existence—and everything else, for that matter) flows independent of, and with no concern for, anything or anyone, but the technique provides the means to work *with* instead of *against* it to a specific end.

The Ch'an approach builds upon the principle that the universe is a stream of Qi, and the individual must navigate that flow. This conception of the universe echoes the Yellow Emperor's theories but with one slight ripple: the meditative act develops the awareness that sparks the change where suffering is transformed into liberation. According to Ch'an, all people possess that awareness, but it is masked by egoistic concerns; or in the words of Bodhidharma: "All mortals have buddha-nature, but it's covered by darkness from which they can't escape. Our buddha-nature is awarness: to be aware and to make others aware. To realize awarness is liberation" (Pine 1987, p.79). The first task is to penetrate this "darkness" and become aware; the second is to help others to become aware.

There is no documentation of Bodhidharma's rationale for how he envisioned Qigong and other Qi work functioning within the practice of cultivating awareness, nor has my own twenty-plus years of formalized training in Buddhism provided any direct answers. Yet this does not invalidate the value of Qi within this tradition; in fact, this gap from the theory of energy to its practice is largely because of a key tenet of Buddhism: Ch'an practice is not prescriptive. The end result is liberation, but there is no set recipe to follow in order to achieve awareness outside of continued work at the meditation techniques. Each person must dedicate himself or herself to the methods in order to discover such liberation individually. Part of that individual discovery is the universality of Qi itself.

If everything is Qi, the act of working with it brings the individual into greater immediacy with things as they are. The Qigong practices attributed to Bodhidharma are vehicles to look inward and see the self as it is—a fluid, flowing energy construct that is shaped by consciousness. The awareness of the foundation of energy alongside the role that the ego mind plays in the construction of the image of a self is the centerpiece of the meditative act. Qi, within this context, is the essential ingredient in the work of liberation: it is the fuel of awareness, and that awareness of the patterns of Qi in the world enable the individual to spark the transformative change from suffering to liberation.

Bodhidharma's teachings of the Eighteen Arhat (Buddha) Hands, which was a predecessor of Shaolin Kung Fu, and the internal Qigong forms of Yi Jin Jing and the Bone, Marrow, and Brain Washing Forms build Qi in the body and mind, that can then be directed to recognizing and navigating the streams of Qi to move toward individual and collective liberation or enlightenment.

The Paths of Qi

Ch'an adheres to the fundamental principles that the Yellow Emperor describes regarding energy, Yin and Yang, and more, but the purpose of using Qi extends beyond health and is cultivated in order to serve the spiritual aim of enlightenment. Ch'an is not unique, though, since Taoism had the same aim long before Bodhidharma or even Buddhism migrated from India to China. It would be remiss not to acknowledge the extent to which Ch'an Buddhism is indebted to Taoism. After all, when Buddhism entered China, it merged with Taoism, and that synthesis was the birth of Ch'an. Without Taoism, there would be no Ch'an Buddhism. There would be other forms, but not Chinese Buddhism. And many of the ideas and techniques of incorporating Qi into meditation and body practices were lifted directly from Taoism. That Ch'an borrowed heavily from Taoism is an open secret, so much so that it is fairly common to find Chinese Buddhist sutras using the word "Tao" to refer to Buddha mind. And not surprisingly, the terms "Tao" and "Buddha mind" are frequently interchanged. The overlap is publicly acknowledged in many sources; for example, *The Book of Balance and Harmony* states:

> *Chan Buddhism, Confucian Noumenalism,*
> *The Taoism of Complete Reality—*
> *Three schools of teaching were set up*
> *To contact later people.*
> *For Buddhists, elements are nonabsolute,*
> *It's necessary to see the essence;*
> *As Confucians investigate phenomena,*
> *They must maintain sincerity.*
> *On the Taoist's alchemical stand*
> *Are kept points of fire;*
> *All kinds of atoms are melted down*
> *In the spiritual mansion.*
> *When you understand all differences*
> *Are resolved in one goal,*
> *Then on the bright terrace*
> *All is spring, inside and out.*
>
> (CLEARY 2003B, P.476)

Taoist master Chang Po-tuan (983–1082 CE), recorded in *Energy, Vitality, Spirit* (1991), points out the shared qualities in this way, which also emphasizes that each branch has the same end:

The Ch'an Master "National Teacher Chung" of the T'ang dynasty caps his recorded sayings with words of Lao Tzu and Chuang-Tzu to reveal the root and branches of the Way. Is it not a fact that the doctrines [of Taoism, Buddhism, and Confucianism] may be three, but the Way is ulitimately one? (Cleary 1991a, p.120)

The Secret of the Golden Flower, a lay manual for Taoist and Buddhist clarifying of the mind, and a cornerstone of Chinese thought, states that the goal of fully actualizing life in Ch'an and Taoism is to develop the same "spiritual pill that gets one out of death and preserves life" (Cleary 1991b, p.46). Even the extremely popular novel, *The Journey to the West*, with the character of the Monkey King, proclaims that "the harmonization of the three schools of Buddhism, Confucianism, and Taoism is a natural thing" (Yu 2006, p.20). And even the Dharma name that I was given when I was fully ordained as a Ch'an Priest acknowledges the dual paths of my own lineage. My name, "Tao-Fa," means the Way (Tao) of the Dharma (Fa), and pays tribute to my Dharma great-grandfather, Holmes Welch (Venerable Shih Mo-Hua), who held lineages in both Taoism and Ch'an. All of these things point to the fact that Ch'an is inseperable from its Taoist roots.

These practices also share the use of Qi within the act of discovering the Way, cultivating the "spiritual pill of life," or discovering "spring inside and out." Taoism (like Ch'an) is not prescriptive, and so much of its practice is obscured in metaphors and indirect poetic language such as "spiritual pill of life" and "spring inside and out." Taoist practice addresses the use of Qi as part of its practice much more explicitly (although masked in allegorical language). For example, *Practical Taoism* states that "the furnace and the cauldron are the body and the mind," which refers—albeit in coded language—to the act of using Qi, and is akin to the Ch'an method of cultivating the physical body (external Kung Fu) and the mind (meditation and Qigong). The Qi of the body must be cultivated and flow smoothly—thereby being the "furnace" of Qi—which is then directed to the mind/cauldron for spiritual cultivation. Body and mind are interdependent and to "affect openness" and manifest perennial spring rests upon the two working together. Taoism refers to this as "dual cultivation," which emphasizes the combination of physiological exercises with mental concentration. A few such methods to meld body and mind can be found throughout Taoist Qigong and Neigong practices, and many of the meditation techniques with names such as Golden Elixir Meditation, Embryonic Breathing, and leading Qi to Shen depend on focusing both body and mind.

Using Qi for spiritual cultivation in Taoism is commonly called "returning to the Source." The methods used are meant to "gather and restore primal energy." One Taoist sage exclaims, "If you want to know the true seed of essence and life, it is nothing but the original, innate, primal, true, unified energy" (Cleary 2003c, p.507). Gathering Qi restores health and initiates a return path to

Wuji, the state of undivided wholesness and balance. The various methods require both the gathering and the refining of Qi, which means that the method is both developing a product (energy) and a process (an energy circuit).

In this way, Qi is both the vehicle and the path. The energy sparks meditative awareness (Shen), which is then channeled into living in accord with the Tao. Such awareness forms a self-reflexive and self-sustaining loop. As the energy is generated, that in turn fuels consciousness, which sparks the ability to *feel*, sense, and experience the Qi, which generates even more energy. The most appropriate analogy to explain this self-reflexive quality is to compare Qi to water. The act of generating Qi is like filling a basin, which is connected to a system of tubes and hoses that attach to other basins. Once the initial basin is filled, the water flows through the tubing and into other basins, which in turn continue flowing into other basins. While the water is flowing through the system, any increase in the pressure of the flow makes it more easy to perceive, feel, recognize, or see that flowing. Like a garden hose, when the water isn't turned on, the hose is limp; when turned on, the force of the water fills the tubing and creates a measurable physical pressure. Returning to the image of Qi, the major Qi reservoir or basin of the body is the Dantian (translated as "Sea of Elixir" or "Energy Seed Field"), which is connected to other reservoirs such as the middle Dantian at the sternum and the upper Dantian in the cerebral cortex through the channels and meridians of the body. Whenever Qi is generated and accumulates at the

Dantian, it flows through the channels, and any increase in the amount of Qi allows for that movement to be more easily discerned or felt. The awareness of the Qi amplifies itself even more and reveals the extent to which the entire system is self-generating and self-reflexive.

The centerpiece of this self-generating and self-sustaining energy system is meditation. The *act* of meditating generates Qi even as the focus of the meditation itself is the sustained awareness, feeling, and consciousness of Qi. Focusing and feeling the Dantian (called Single-Pointed Meditation) is one such meditation where concentration is maintained by focusing on one spot or "point." Once the Qi is generated, focused awareness can direct the Qi. This is the essence of a range of Taoist meditative and Qigong practices such as Small Circulation (or Microcosmic) Breathing, or Embryonic Mediation. In all cases, the intentional mind (Yi) leads the Qi. Awareness of the Qi and the play of Yin and Yang within the body is extended outward to see the balancing and harmonizing of Qi that is the flow of the world at large. Energy is not only generated but is also meant to be used to cultivate a broader awareness.

The Taoist perspective of enlightenment is to affect openness in order to return to the Source. Taoist practice seeks to not resist the Way of the Tao and to be in accord with the stream of Qi. Lao Tzu refers to this as the way of "unimpeded harmony," and attainment of this state depends on "nondoing": "Do nondoing...strive for nonstriving" (Cleary 1992, p.48). Essentially the self that is preoccupied with fame, power, and materiality gets in the way. To "strive for nonstriving" is to remove the impediments that obstruct the self from being open. *Taoist Meditation*, an important Taoist collection of writings, describes this process as one of increased intimacy and spontaneity: "The work of learning the way requires greater intimacy with each passing day, greater intimacy with each passing hour. Eventually you develop spontaneous familiarity and unite with the way" (Cleary 2000, p.68). The intimacy is both internal—to "know thyself" in the famous words of Socrates—and external, which shapes the nature of the individual's interaction with the world. This "spontaneous familiarity" is the heart of nondoing and nonstriving, and is called Wu wei, which is often translated as "doing nothing." Wu wei is not apathy; rather, the concept refers to the ability to respond appropriately to a given situation, and by responding appropriately, interfering as little as possible with the Tao.

To act in harmony is not to resist the flow of the Tao and to abide in the present situation. Such "nonresistance" is not passive since action may be required. For example, if a person witnesses a wrong being commited (such as a crime of violence or theft), "spontaneous familiarity" would translate as taking action in some way that responds appropriately and seeks to correct a situation, whether personally involving oneself to stop the crime or alerting the authorities. Wu wei is acting in a way that is not founded upon one's own "striving" for fame, recognition, and power, but rather seeks to reestablish a correct balance. The emotions of greed, anger, fear, and desire are exactly the contrived self-centered flaws that interfere with the Tao and block the individual from returning to the Source—and those emotions and self-centeredness are often the catalysts for unethical if not criminal behavior. The purpose is to return to simplicity and the authentic self, called P'u in Taoism (the uncarved block of the real self), which is absent of desire, anger, and greed. As Lao Tzu writes:

I have three treasures
That I keep and hold:
One is mercy,
The second is frugality,
The third is not presuming
To be at the head of the world.
By reason of mercy,
One can be brave.
By reason of frugality,
One can be broad.
By not presuming
To be at the head of the world,
One can make your potential last.

(CLEARY 1992, P.52)

The ability to act in accord with the Tao—to be merciful, frugal, and humble—grows from the act of looking inward, turning the "gaze around," and then allowing that more authentic self to respond appropriately and spontaneously. That act is the product of meditative conception that rests upon Qi. As Zhang Sanfeng, the famous Taoist monk credited with the creation of Taiji, once wrote: "Accumulating vitality is setting up the foundation" (Cleary 2000, p.129). Energy is cultivated and then directed to increase Shen, and that heightened awareness provides a more broad and less egocentric perspective that allows a person to act with greater intimacy with the moment, and have access to an even more deep stream of Qi. The return to the Source is a returning to the simplicity of the self that is beyond the human foibles of greed, ego, and desire, and that process leads to Wu wei—of being in the immediacy of the Tao, which helps to preserve the essence of energy, vitality, and spirit.

The Qi of the Immortal Moment

All of these techniques included in Buddhism, Taoism, and Traditional Chinese Medicine share two specific goals: first, to recognize the various aspects of Qi in the self and in the universe, which can be discerned in the play of Yin and Yang or through the Five Elements Theory; and second, to master the process of generating and directing Qi in order to reestablish the original, primal energy. For the Yellow Emperor, that returning to the Source is being simple and living in harmony with the Tao, which is the key to health and long life. For Ch'an Buddhism, it is to awaken the Buddha mind and achieve liberation from all that is not the Tao; for Taoism, it is drawing upon the primal energy that creates balance and allows entry into the Tao. Each of these practices share the belief that Qi is universal and its rule applies to the general and the specific. Patterns of Qi can be discerned and discovered within the self and the world. And finally, those patterns of Qi can be harnassed to serve the purposes of health, healing, well-being, and spiritual enlightenment.

These traditions paint rich depictions of what it means to reach these higher stages of health, well-being, and spiritual awakening. The Yellow Emperor describes a life of peace, calm, and a long healthy life:

> The sages lived peacefully under heaven on earth, following the rhythms of the planet and the universe. They adapted to society without being swayed by cultural trends. They were free from emotional extremes and lived a balanced, contented existence. Their outward appearance, behavior, and thinking did not reflect the conflicting norms of society. The sages appeared busy but were never depleted. Internally they did not overburden themselves. They abided in calmness, recognizing the empty nature of phenomenological existence. The sages lived over one hundred years because they did not scatter and disperse their energies. (Ni 1995, p.27)

Similarly, Lao Tzu describes moments of divine stillness and oneness with the Tao:

Attain the climax of emptiness,
Preserve the utmost quiet:
As myraid things act in concert,
I thereby observe the return.
Things flourish,
Then each returns to its root.
Returning to the root is called stillness:
Stillness is called return to Life,
Return to Life is called the constant,
Knowing the constant is called enlightenment.

...

This Way is everlasting,
Not endangered by physical death.

(CLEARY 1992, P.18)

The sages of Taoism—who are referred to as "Real Humans"—are often called Immortals "not endangered by physical death." *The Book of Balance and Harmony* speaks of achieving a state of perpetual spring—"inside and out"— that is beyond the reach of aging and decay. And Ch'an Buddhism has as its goal that the fully awakened person achieve nirvana and transcend mortality.

The promise of immortality is intertwined with the paths of these practices, and using Qi properly is the key to reach this hallowed end.

The next three chapters on Body, Breath, and Mind/ Heart, respectively, discuss in more detail the various techniques of generating Qi, all of which come together in the final chapter which includes a range of time tested exercises, Qigong, and meditations. I make no promises that the person who incorporates these exercises into a daily regime will become an "immortal" and live forever as a result. Nor is my goal here to refute or affirm the possibility of immortality. And yet, if immortality is thought of not as a limitless quantity of living years but as a broader and richer quality of life, these practices open onto the immortality of each moment. After all, if we are healthy and without pain, disease, and suffering, if we are calm and contented with our lives, if we have discovered an inner value that gives shape and purpose to all that we do, and if our hearts and minds are at ease, we achieve a lasting sense of peace, abundance, and depth that reveals the richness of the moment. From that persective we recognize the work of the Tao and allow ourselves to abide in the flow of immortal Qi. We find within ourselves the Sage, the Buddha, the Immortal, the Real Human, and we return peacefully to the Source.

CHAPTER 3

Opening the Energy Gates of the Body

My student Stacey stood at the entrance to the studio with something unrecognizable in her hands. From the way that she was holding her body—shifting her weight back and forth, the slight tension in her shoulders, and looking around her with fleeting glances—something was afoot. As I drew closer, I realized that she held a present wrapped in festive paper. With a smirk on her face, she handed the package to me with a cry of "Happy birthday, Sensei!" I eagerly tore open the box. Inside was a gold t-shirt with sayings from the original 1984 *Karate Kid* printed on it. The front of the shirt had an image of the teacher from the Cobra Kai Academy saying "Bow to your sensei." The back of the shirt had "Fear does not exist in the dojo" printed in big black letters. Stacey and I laughed. Hard. And I told her how much I loved her present. The irony of the gift was not lost on me since everything about it—the language of "sensei" and "dojo" and the messages—stands in direct contrast with the essence of Chinese Internal Arts. The t-shirt was not the only time Stacey would poke me jokingly. Sometimes in class she would call me "Sensei" instead of the traditional "Sifu" and say things like "pain is weakness leaving the body" and "pain is temporary," not so much to be a smart aleck but because the sayings conflicted with the core of the Internal Arts that I frequently repeated: relax; listen to your body; if something hurts, we need to address it; and don't overdo it. Stacey's joking set a playful tone of fellowship for the classes, but the main reason I allowed it was because the jokes demonstrated an oppositional understanding that highlighted how the essence of the Internal Arts differs in many ways from Western approaches to the body and exercise.

The principles of Taiji and Qigong contrast with many of the prevailing workout attitudes of the West with its mantra of "No Pain, No Gain," which is usually accompanied by images of people panting, grimacing, and sweating. The contemporary exercise methods of pushing harder *and* faster *and* longer might be effective ways to build muscle strength, increase cardiovascular health, and burn calories, but in terms of Qi, such approaches consume more energy than that which is generated and are counterindicative to the foundation of many Traditional Chinese Medicine principles as espoused by the Yellow Emperor. Since the methodologies of Western exercise are not built upon Traditional Chinese Medicine theory, the body is not conceived as an energy system, and the benefits associated with the Internal Arts are noticeably absent.

Master Yang Yang, a delightful and expansive Taiji and Qigong teacher, plays off of this Western mantra when he exclaims that the appropriate slogan for the Internal Arts is "No Pain, More Gain." Pain is not efficient when it comes to energy since it uses and restricts the flow of Qi. The natural response to pain is tightness and impeded circulatory flow, either through muscle constriction or inflammation at a site of injury. Even the thought of pain can prompt tightness. Observing another person fall down and get hurt can trigger a physical response for some people. Contemporary psychology calls this response synesthesia for pain built upon a mirror system where the pain is reflected from the person who experiences it to the person who observes and absorbs it. Whether it is a pain that we ourselves experience or we observe in others, the physical response to pain is an impediment to the circulatory system and the Qi pathways of the body.

The absence of pain—and the concomitant absence of tightness of the body—allows the body to heal and strengthen itself, which is the gist of Yang Yang's "No Pain, More Gain." Simply put, the state of the body—whether it is relaxed or tight, its structure, and whether it is rooted or not—directly impacts the quantity and quality of Qi. Learning how to regulate the body is necessary to working with Qi. To maximize the health of the body and to harness Qi, three interrelated physical qualities are necessary: Song (the principle of the body being calm and relaxed), structure (the body adheres to proper alignment for open circulation), and rootedness (the body sinks and creates a foundation). The fundamental technique that unites these three qualities is feeling.

Bow to Your Senses

When I wrote to Stacey to tell her that I was using the story of her gift in my analysis of the principle of the body and Qi, the word "Sensei" kept getting changed to "Senses" in my messages. At first, I was irritated but amused by having to type and retype "Sensei" as if Stacey was continuing to taunt me from beyond the keyboard. But then it struck me how profoundly appropriate the message was. "Bow to your senses." And this message echoes one of Grandmaster Helen Wu's frequent refrains: "Listen to your body." We need to spend more time listening to our bodies. Our senses reveal the body to us, and they are the vehicles of our consciousness. When we bow to our senses, we are honoring the pathways to feel and work with our physical body and beyond. In fact, the senses are our means of perception, and, to borrow the famous phrase from the poet William Blake, bowing to them "cleanses the doors of perception" (Erdman 1988). The complete lines from his "The Marriage of Heaven and Hell" are extremely relevant: "If the doors of perception were cleansed everything would appear to man as it is: infinite. ... For man has closed himself up, till he sees all things thro' narrow chinks of his cavern" (p.39). The senses can open onto the infinite—the Tao—or, like Plato's famous allegory of the cave, they can reveal a small narrow view of shadows that are mistaken for the real.

Parallel to Blake's concept that man has "closed himself off" and perceives the world through a narrow view, Buddhism and Taoism often refer to the five senses as thieves since sensory attention is often directed outward—to look at or listen to something external—instead of turning that gaze and ear inward toward the internal landscape. The doors of perception disperse Qi if the senses are used in a haphazard way that constantly flits here and there like a butterfly seemingly without intention and focus. That outward attention leads the self to latch onto external things. Energy and attention is further dispersed into the emotional attachments of those things and the strategizing of how to obtain them: I like that; I want that: How do I get that? Yet those same thieves are the tools that bring us into our bodies and into an intimate awareness of Qi. The goal is not to negate the senses—a point of misunderstanding for many newcomers to meditation who think that mediation is zoning out—but to fine-tune the senses for the purpose of deeper feeling. One of the classic sayings is that we should look inward three times a day. The senses are the means to examine, explore, and feel the body and its Qi. "When the light is turned around," according to the author of *The Secret of the Golden Flower*, "the energies of heaven and earth, yin and yang, all congeal" (Cleary 1991b, p.17). The act of "looking" at the body is an inward turning that allows us to feel and perceive the self. The ultimate goal of the Internal Arts is "feeling": the body, its pathways and circulation, its health and well-being. To develop health and power depends on the ability to discern the internal landscape of the body and the streaming flow of its Qi. Learning how to listen to the body and then adjusting its state, structure, and rootedness appropriately is the path to harnessing and using Qi.

Yet to what exactly are we listening? What does Qi feel like? The answers to these questions drive at the heart of Qi itself.

The Qi Furnace

The body itself is composed of two major kinds of Qi: prenatal Qi, which is inherited from parents; and postnatal Qi, which is obtained from external sources such as food and air. The Qi of body can manifest as a number of sensations such as warmth (Yang Qi), fullness, heaviness, magnetic polarity, electric currents, or as a cool, menthol feeling (Yin Qi).[2] The body stores, processes, circulates, generates, and ultimately uses Qi. It is the system of channels, pathways, meridians, organs, and vessels through which Qi moves; and along with the mind and the spirit, the body is nourished and sustained by Qi and will perish without it. The body has three major Qi reservoirs, which are called Dantians—the lower (real), middle (sternum), and upper Dantian (middle of the cerebral cortex)—with the most significant one being the lower or real Dantian (Sea of Elixir, or Energy Seed Field), which is about one inch below the navel and toward the center of the body.

Being able to properly locate and feel the lower Dantian is absolutely crucial to working with the body's energy.

One technique to help locate this Dantian uses the abdominal muscles in conjunction with the breath to create an internal pressure that emphasizes the Qi of the Dantian. To perform this exercise, stand with the arms loosely at the side of the body or sit in a chair without touching the back of the chair and with the hands resting on the thighs with the palms facing downward. Inhale slowly and deeply through the nose while simultaneously drawing the abdominal muscles inward. Gently hold the breath with the abdominal muscles contracted for a few seconds,[3] then exhale again through the nose and release the abdominal muscles. Repeat the exercise a few times to intensify the effect. Pay attention to any sensations that occur in the lower abdomen since the site of those sensations is the Dantian. As this practice is refined and honed, this exercise may generate a feeling of fullness, warmth, or pressure (even slight discomfort) in the Dantian. Accompanying any feeling in the Dantian may be a sensation of warmth that extends outward to the Five Gates—the palms of the hands (Laogong, or Labor Palace Cavity), the balls of the feet (Yongquan Cavity, or Bubbling Well), and the crown of the head (Baihui, or Heaven's Cap). This warmth housed in the Dantian that spreads through the body and into the limbs prompted ancient Taoist sources to refer to the body as the furnace, which is an extremely apt analogy since the body is both the structure as well as the means to generate, process, and refine Qi, which sustains life.

Regardless of our effort or consciousness of Qi, the furnace works with or without our attention, but there are techniques that make the generation and circulation of Qi more efficient. These methods enhance both the ability to cultivate and refine Qi. The principles of Relaxation, Structure, and Rooting have been used for hundreds if not thousands of years to increase the generation of energy in the Dantian and fuel the body as a whole The classic saying is that when the body is tense, the Qi is tense. When the Qi is tense, the harmony is disrupted, which can lead to illness and disease. Muscular constriction restricts the Qi channels of the body, and any impediment creates an imbalance throughout the entire body.

The first step is to relax. Relaxation, though, is not a passive activity like sleeping or zoning out. The common perception is that relaxation is sleep, and for many beginning practitioners of seated meditation or recumbent Qigong exercises, when the body relaxes, they fall asleep. Closing the eyes prompts the person to shut down conscious activity and fall asleep. But during sleep, the mind is not gazing inward in an act of self-reflexive or heightened consciousness; rather, the mind is in a dream state while unconsciously maintaining organ function. Sleeping is detached and unguided. The method of relaxation that applies to the life of Qi is active—aware, concentrated, and focused—not in a furrowed-brow way but rather in a broad and inclusive perception that is conscious of both internal and external processes. The Chinese word for this form of relaxation is Song, which might best be translated as "at ease."

The term has military connotations of a soldier standing "at ease," and if Song is placed within such a context, its active character is evident. When a soldier stands at attention, the body and the mind are rigid with muscles and concentration engaged in a position that is demanding and utilizes a great deal of energy to maintain. The position of "at ease" releases the muscles into a more comfortable stance that can be held for a much greater period of time and is much less energy-draining. The concentration, similarly, is looser as well, although awareness is maintained in order to respond quickly to any given commands. The essence of Song is a soft, relaxed body accompanied with the heart and mind at ease and unburdened by tension, distraction, and distress. When such distractions are eliminated, the body, mind, and heart are unified into an undisrupted whole.

Relaxation opens awareness to the present moment. Contemporary Western philosophy refers to this as bringing the self fully into Being. The elimination (or reduction) of tension—physical, emotional, and intellectual—lifts the obstacles that veil the present moment. After all, worry and anxiety is a projection into an unknown future and what might happen; continuous sadness and regret is a fixation upon an unchangeable past. Song requires a letting go and a release. Relaxing is not a passive act but one that requires an awareness and a monitoring of tightness and tension in the body as well as an identification of the sources or triggers—whether they are the result of a physical condition, disease, illness, or injury, or are the outward manifestations of the internal self and its stress, anxiety, fear, sadness or other emotional or psychological conditions. The qualities of the mind and heart and their relationship to Qi is the focus of Chapter 5, but suffice it to say for now that the state of the mind and heart are interwoven with the condition of the body and are not separate states. For the body to be relaxed requires that the mind and heart be at ease, and vice versa. The body is the foundation for the mind, heart, breath, and Qi, and the efficiency of each of these aspects rests upon the principle of Song.

The releasing of physical tension allows for the greater circulation of Qi. When the body is tense, the Qi is tense. When the Qi is tense, it is more difficult to feel its circulation and thereby regulate it. Any muscular constriction or impediment is like a stream littered with debris: the blockage impedes the flow of water, creating a dam that will escalate into further blockages. Tightness within the body impedes the path of Qi. To demonstrate, from a seated position, turn an arm so that the palm is resting face up upon the thigh. Relax the arm and observe the coloration of the palm. Now close the hand into a tight fist and hold that position. Notice how the color around the knuckles and the exposed fingers grows paler as the blood circulation is obstructed by the tightness of the fist. Then open and relax the fist and observe the circulation and color return to the palm and fingers. Tension restricts; relaxation opens. The goal is to achieve a state of Song from head to feet. The feeling is like standing in a warm shower. As the water flows down from the head to the face, neck, and shoulders, allow each part of the body to let go of any tightness. Then extend this process of releasing into the torso—relaxing the chest, ribs, and diaphragm. The back softens at the base of the neck, between the shoulder blades, and then the lower back. The waist and then hips release any tightness, which allows the thighs, knees, and then ankles to relax. The flow of warm water envelopes the entire body until all tension, discomfort, and resistance is dissolved. The goal (in the words of the Taoist saying) is to "be like water" since water is without tension, hardness, and is not bothered when confronted by an obstacle; or as Lao Tzu remarks, "Higher good is like water [because it moves] without contention" (Cleary 1992, p.12). The physical body should be unobstructed and open, and to be unencumbered allows the heart and mind to be free of contention.

Any physical tightness, from the seemingly insignificant to the most extreme and painful, creates blockages and constriction. Softening the body smoothes out the circulation and allows for heightened self-awareness. Relaxation is softness, which allows for the flow of blood and Qi to be unimpeded and enables the body to balance itself. The same softness opens awareness so that it can penetrate past the tightness of muscular constriction and into the deeper recesses of the body in order to feel Qi more acutely. This principle should be evident from the earlier exercise of finding and feeling the Dantian by holding and releasing the abdominal muscles. The Dantian is not readily felt when holding the breath and clenching the muscles. Muscular tightness obscures the deeper feeling. Only when the breath and muscles are released does the circulation open and the sensations of the Dantian can be discerned. Similarly, a relaxed body allows for the discovery of other pockets of tension, and once those are identified, even deeper Song takes place. The entire process perpetually increases sensitivity for experiencing deeper relaxation and circulation by identifying problem areas and learning how to release any tightness, all of which allows feeling to extend even farther into the body.

Softening the body triggers a sinking of weight as well. When the body relaxes, weight flows to the ground. In effect, relaxing prompts the body to root. As each portion of the body softens from the head downward, the muscles relax and the joints open, and the feeling is one in which the weight of the body pushes into the ground. The word "rooting" suggests an insightful parallel with trees. For most trees, the root ball (that which is underground and supports the remainder of the tree) is equal in size to the tree's canopy spread against the sky. The roots are an inverted mirror of the canopy of branches. The roots underground and the branches above are balanced and even, and if it is not, the tree is in danger of being toppled in a storm or over time. When the body is rooted, it is as if a mirror image of the self extends from the feet and into the ground.

Rooting relaxes the body into the earth, and like a tree, that root is strengthened through the proper structuring of the body, which also facilitates the unrestricted circulation of Qi. Rooting allows for the pulsing of Qi through the body; the proper structure enables Qi to circulate freely.

An Iron Rod Wrapped in Silk

The rich writings of internal martial artists and especially Taiji masters provides an invaluable framework to understand the significant role that physical structure plays for Qi. The classic treatises on Taiji outline numerous principles regarding the proper structure of the body and its alignment. While these writings cross various differing styles, one tenet is shared: the correct stance of the body provides the architectural framework that maximizes Song, Rooting, and Qi circulation. In these traditions, one of the recurring stances is named "Wuji" or "no polarities," which means that the whole body is in harmony, without Yin and Yang, or substantial or insubstantial qualities. Granted, to be without oppositional polarities may be an unattainable ideal; nevertheless, the concept of Wuji frames a fundamental goal of the self—to seek balance and harmony within, which begins with a balanced physical exterior. A brief sketch of these Internal Arts principles offers valuable pointers to proper stance and structure:[4]

- The body should be aligned vertically forming the "Standing Pole."

- The neck and head are aligned with the spine, and the top of the head should feel as if it is suspended by a thread from above. Draw the head up from inside the body.

- Sink the chest and raise the back.

- Relax the shoulders and sink the elbows.

- Relax the waist and hips; the Kua or bridge of the hips should be open.

- The knees are open (slightly bent) and the lower abdomen is relaxed.

- Draw the tailbone up.

- No tilting or leaning in the posture; maintain the integrity of the standing pole.

To align the neck and spine and bring the entire body into position, two sayings are useful pointers. The first saying is "Imagine that you are one inch taller." The second saying is "Without turning your head, listen behind you." These two sayings refine the standing pole and harmonize the whole. When all of these principles are united, the Qi sinks to the Dantian naturally and without effort. In addition, the pathway from Dantian to middle and upper Dantians (sternum and cerebral cortex) is unobstructed. Each of these guiding structural principles impacts the circulation of Qi throughout the eight channels of the body (Figure 3.1).

The previous chapter (Chapter 2) discusses the eight channels of the body as well as the organ pathways in light of Traditional Chinese Medicine as well as Five Elements Theory. These channels form a series of gates and rivers that facilitate the circulation of Qi throughout the body as a whole. Briefly, the body is composed of eight major channels that are interconnected much like a series of intersecting roads:

- The Governing Channel runs from the Dantian downward, between the legs to Huiyin, and then up the back to finish above the upper lip at Renzhong (acupressure point GV 26).

- The Conception Channel starts at the bottom lip and moves downward to the Dantian. The Conception Channel forms a loop with the Governing Channel into what is known as the Microcosmic Orbit.[5]

- The Thrusting Channel goes from Huiyin (between the legs) to the Baihui—Heaven's Cap at the crown of the head.

- The Belt Channel circles the waist and crosses the Governing Channel at the Mingmen (Life's Gate) and the Conception Channel at the front of the Dantian (sometimes referred to as the False Dantian).

- The outside of the legs is the Yang Leg Channel which runs down to the heel, and the inside of the legs running upward is the Yin Leg Channel.

• The outside of the arms is the Yang Arm Channel which runs down to the palm, and the inside of the arms running upward is the Yin Arm Channel.

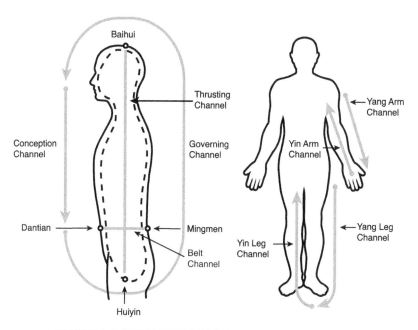

FIGURE 3.1 EIGHT ENERGETIC CHANNELS OF THE BODY

When the eight channels are overlaid with the structure principles, the integral relation between body position and Qi circulation is evident.

The emphasis upon the Standing Pole of the Body, the alignment of neck and head in relation to the spine, and the feeling that the top of the head is suspended from above as if by a thread opens the Thrusting and the Governing channels. Furthermore, the alignment of the back enables the three gates—the lower back (Mingmen/ Life's Gate), middle of the back (between the shoulder blades), and the neck (Jade Pillow) to be unobstructed so that the Qi smoothly flows from the Dantian to the upper Dantian. The body tilting or leaning forward or back pinches these channels and hampers the flow. Two other structural principles also impact the flow of Qi through the Governing and Conception channels. Sinking the chest (allowing the sternum to slightly hollow) stretches open the Governing Channel (making it Yang) while relaxing the Conception Channel (making it Yin) allowing for the Qi to circulate up the back and down the front in what is known as the Microcosmic Orbit. The slight drawing up of the tailbone decreases any resistance through the lower portion of the Microcosmic Orbit—that is, from Dantian through Huiyin (between the genitals and the anus) and to the Mingmen. A relaxed waist further contributes to the circulation through the Microcosmic Orbit as well as the pathway through the Belt Channel connecting Mingmen and Dantian. Not coincidentally, the emphasis upon the open rotation of the waist in Taiji not only is important for generating power but also stimulates the Belt Channel and activates Wei qi, the protective Qi of the immune system.

Lastly, the emphasis upon the shoulders and elbows being relaxed and the hips and knees open engages the energetic channels of the arms and legs. Any tightness in the joints—shoulders, elbows, wrists, hips, knees, or ankles—hampers circulation into the limbs. Because of the intimate connection between the joints, any tightness in one joint also causes tightness elsewhere. These joints are known as the three unities—or sometimes the three brothers and sisters—wherein the shoulders are related to the hips, the elbows to the knees, and the wrists to the ankles. If one joint is tight, its counterpart is tense as well. To demonstrate, try this simple exercise: From a standing position relax both the knees and the elbows, then lock only the elbows. Feel how the body unconsciously tenses the knees as well; or feel the awkwardness when the knees are locked and the elbows open, and vice versa. Any tension in the elbows is transferred to the knees. Similarly, the same intimate internal relationship holds for the shoulders and hips as well as the wrists and ankles. Relaxed shoulders and elbows translate into the channels of the arms and legs being fully opened, thereby allowing Qi to circulate into the limbs and, ultimately, to be incorporated into various movements. When the joints are open, Qi can easily flow to the Five Gates of the palms, feet, and crown of the head. The unobstructed flow of Qi to the palms is particularly important in developing Fajin—striking force—wherein energy is converted to Jin.[6]

Overall, the Eight Extraordinary Channels form a network that includes the entire body, which is why certain leg movements, for example, are effective for headaches since the channels of the legs can reach the neck and brain.[7] The emphasis upon proper posture in meditation practices—whether seated or standing— relates to the circulation of Qi so that the flow can reach the Dantian or upper Dantian for spiritual cultivation. These physiological principles serve two purposes: first, the proper alignment and structure of the body minimizes physical strain and contributes to a state of attentive relaxation or Song; and second, the correct stance enables the Qi to flow unimpeded throughout the body and its channels. Song and stance are interwoven tools for the circulation, and harmonization of Qi, stance, and Song, from the perspective of Martial Arts training, translates into a relaxed body capable of moving quickly without compromising foundation or Root. An individual is able to respond (defensively or offensively) with quickness and force, and the unobstructed flow of Qi allows for the tapping of "Jin" or energetic power. The core (stance) is firm and rooted; the muscles, tendons, and joints are relaxed and soft. The combination of Song and stance allows for the Qi to move smoothly through the body and for energy to be directed to the limbs and gates—all of which is alluded to in the famous saying that the body in Taiji is an Iron Rod Wrapped in Silk: a body that is solid and relaxed, rooted and flexible, Yin and Yang, active and aware.

Stoking the Fire

Paying attention to body structure and Song is akin to carefully building a fire. If the wood is seasoned and arranged in such a way that the fire can "breath," the fire will light and burn more efficiently. While the fire of Qi is always lit—at least while a person still lives—that fire can be managed, stoked, and controlled for the preservation of life. An efficient Qi system is founded upon rootedness and relaxation whereby the circulation can be amplified and directed through the movement of the body and the mind. When the circulation is smooth and balanced, the body reaches what is known as Wu Qi Chao Yuan, or "Five Qis toward their origins," which regulates the organs and prevents disease. To return Qi to the organs and bolster health builds upon the direct stimulation of the organs as well as the body's twelve primary channels that are related to an organ (Figure 3.2). Those organs and their respective channels are:

- Lung (Yin Channel)

- Large Intestine (Yang Channel)

- Stomach (Yang Channel)

- Spleen (Yin Channel)

- Heart (Yin Channel)

- Small Intestine (Yang Channel)

- Bladder (Yang Channel)

- Kidney (Yin Channel)

- Pericardium (Yin Channel)

- Triple Burner (Yang Channel)

- Gall Bladder (Yang Channel)

- Liver (Yin Channel).

These channels may be more easily envisioned from the chart used by acupuncture wherein the map of the body is shown as organ pathways with seamlessly connected channels.

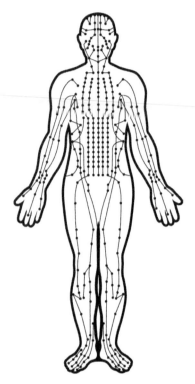

FIGURE 3.2 THE ORGAN CHANNELS OF THE BODY AS DEPICTED IN A TYPICAL ACUPUNCTURE CHART

Even though the Heart Channel is not directly attached to the Kidney, for example, the path from the Heart connects to the Small Intestine, which flows into the Bladder, and then to the Kidney. The whole body is a seamless circuit, and any blockage, excess, or diminishment of circulation at one point can impact all of the other parts.[8]

Direct stimulation of the body's eight Energetic Channels or twelve Primary Channels helps to regulate and harmonize the circulation of Qi. The classic saying is that Yi (mind intention) leads Qi. Where the mind goes, the Qi follows. Yet physical stimulation pumps Qi throughout the body, and a focused and directed movement has the capacity to target a specific channel or organ. The fundamental physiological principle is that Qi can be directed to a specific energetic channel or to a particular organ by bending, stretching, and massaging that site or path. For example, extending the chin forward stretches and activates the Conception Channel that runs down the front of the torso, and then withdrawing the chin into the chest "bends" the same channel. The movement targets and pumps Qi to the specific part of the body utilized in the physical movement. In the same way, rounding the shoulders forward and arching the back stretches the Governing Channel and activates it (making it "Yang") while the hollowed chest and the Conception Channel become "Yin." Coordinating this movement with inhalation and exhalation adds diaphragmatic pressure that internally stimulates and massages the engaged channels more. The arching of the back and chest (which along with the spine, arms, and legs constitute the "five bows" of the body) gathers and releases the Qi through the body thereby expressing Qi through the physical action. The same principle of movement can be applied to targeting a particular organ and its corresponding channels as well. These principles are the foundation of therapeutic and health Qigong wherein the sequence of movements activates Qi.

Bend Stretch Massage

The Five Animals Sport or Frolic (Wu Qin Xi) is one of the best examples of how a dynamic movement can be used to activate a specific channel. The Qigong form consists of five sets of five movements, each of which corresponds to an organ. Tiger/Liver; Deer/Kidney; Bear/Spleen; Monkey/Heart; and Crane/Lung. The form in its entirety works through the five Yin or Zang organs and their corresponding Yang or Fu organs by repeating a set of moves. Traditionally each animal has five steps, totaling twenty-five movements for the entire set. Deer, for example, corresponds to Kidney. Throughout the set for Deer, the lower rib area of the back, where the kidneys are located, is the center radial point for each of the movements. Each bend and stretch and the consummate physical action begins and/or returns to the site of the kidneys providing continuous direct stimulation to the organs and their respective channels.

Pawing the Ground, usually the second in the sequence of five Deer movements, illustrates how bending, stretching, and massaging the kidneys work in relation to the action of the body and breath. To start Deer Paws the Ground, extend the left foot forward and the right foot back in a classic bow stance.[9] Both hands remain in loose fists with the palm sides of the fists facing downward and the knuckles upward forming deer "hooves" with the hands. The arm of the left fist is extended straight forward at shoulder height, and directly above the left knee. The arm of the right fist is extended straight back. The lower back along the ribs will be stretched from the stance and arm position alone (Figure 3.3).

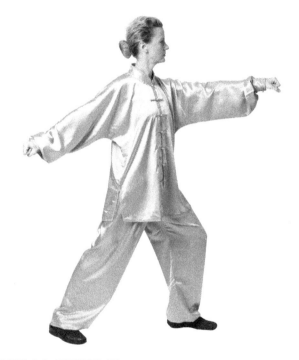

FIGURE 3.3 OPENING STANCE FOR DEER PAWS THE GROUND

To execute the movement, simultaneously turn the waist and rotate the upper body to the right, shift the weight onto the right foot, and draw the left fist backward toward the right shoulder. Inhale as the weight shifts onto the right leg and the fist is brought to the shoulder (Figure 3.4).

The right fist then smoothly drops to waist level and the weight shifts back to the right foot as the waist turns back to front, which leads the right fist forward and up to the starting position (Figure 3.4).

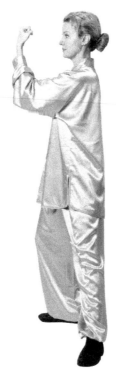

FIGURE 3.4 TURNING THE BODY AND SHIFTING WEIGHT FOR DEER PAWS THE GROUND

Exhale with the "pawing" forward motion (Figure 3.5). The entire process rotates on the kidneys, alternating bending and stretching the left and right sides, and the breathing creates an internal pressure that pushes and releases with the move. The angle of the pressure changes, pushes, and releases throughout creating an undulating pump upon the kidneys, their channel, as well as the Belt Channel.

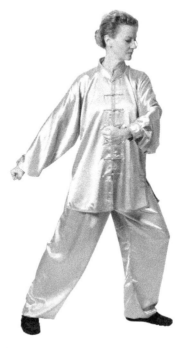

FIGURE 3.5 ROTATING THE ARM AND FIST TO PAW THE GROUND

Focus is maintained upon the kidneys throughout the physical action in order to ensure that the movement targets the respective organ. In addition, the mind monitors that the body remains soft and relaxed. Any muscular tightness acts like a shield that does not allow the movement to penetrate past the surface and to reach the internal organ. If the joints of the arms are locked and muscles clenched in the above Pawing the Ground, for example, the diaphragmatic pressure from the breath stays higher in the chest and does not reach the kidneys. Moreover, such tightness will pump Qi into the muscles and divert energy from the internal organs and diffuse the energy outward. The purpose of the external physical action is to generate and stimulate the internal processes of the organs and channels for health and healing.

In order to maximize the internal work, Qigong approaches physical structure as a tool to engage and activate specific areas of the body. For that reason, the standing pole in Qigong isn't as rigorously maintained as in Taiji since a person may need to lean forward—thereby "breaking" the standing pole of the body—in order to stimulate a specific energetic channel or to create pressure upon an organ. The movements do not need to adhere to the same structural integrity since the "opponent" in Qigong is illness and any vulnerability created by improper stance does not have the same repercussions as a martial artist would have against another person. Although Qigong itself is not martial in nature, there are forms such as Iron Shirt (Tie Bu Shan) or Golden Bell Cover (Jing Zhong Zhao) that strengthen specific parts of body by leading Qi to specific parts of the body. Instead of the Qi directed to an organ for health and healing, the structure of the body and Song is utilized to focus Qi to an area to protect the body or to create power. Yet even in those martial Qigong techniques, the same principle applies of using the posture and breath to power and direct Qi.

Using the Fire of Qi

The Internal Martial Arts emphasis upon structure and Song has to do with the generation of power. Yang Cheng-Fu, the patriarch of modern Yang-style Taiji, explained that "If you cannot relax and sink [root], the two shoulders will be raised up and tense. The qi will follow them and the whole body cannot get power" (Wile 1983, p.12). Rooting and relaxation directly impact power and the individual's ability to access Qi. Furthermore, a movement uses the channels to lead Qi through the body and transform it into Jin. For example, a traditional Yang-style Taiji posture, such as Ward-off (Peng), engages the bow of the back and the chest, thereby activating the Governing and Conception channels. Furthermore, the bowing movement pumps and releases the front and back of the lungs as well—delivering and directing Qi into the action of the arms.

Sun Lu Tang, the great Baguazhang and Hsing-I master and creator of Sun-style Taiji, understood explicitly how changes in body position can be used to alter the flow and nature of Qi. San Ti (Trinity Posture) is the centerpiece of Sun-style training as well as Chen Standing Meditation.[10] Traditionally the posture is executed by assuming a bow stance with 60 percent of the body's weight on the back foot and 40 percent forward (Figure 3.6). Whichever leg is forward, that side arm is extended outward at shoulder-socket height, and the opposite arm is slightly bent so that the hand is near the opposite elbow in what is known as "Palm Chasing Elbow."[11]

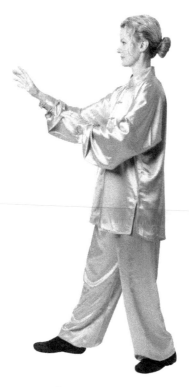

FIGURE 3.6 CLASSIC SAN TI POSTURE

Sun's earlier version of San Ti had both hands palms down with fingers extended forward. Later, he modified the hand position so that the finger pointed upward in the classic "Tiger's Mouth" position. The difference in the hand position was an explicit response to his understanding of Qi circulation and how that Qi was to be used. Sun Jian Yun, Sun's daughter, explained in *Xing Yi Quan Xue* (Miller 1993) that her father changed the hand position in order to accommodate cultivating or emitting Qi either for improving health or for fighting:

He felt that when the hand was held straight out the Qi was projected from the hand. He said this was good for fighting, but was not good for cultivation. When cultivating Qi, one should keep the Qi in the body. When the hand is held up, the Qi is held in the hand. (p.44)

The hand position not only alters the generation and circulation of the Qi, but also whether the Qi is moving out from the person or is retained within. Sun Lu Tang understood how the structure of the posture enhances the energy of the martial applications and allows for the expression of energy through the movements and postures.[12] For the same reason, the classic Taiji slogan is that the chest should be slightly convex in order to store (and not emit) Qi from the middle Dantian. When the chest bows outward, the energy is projected forward and outward. Structural changes in body position—even small ones such as hand placement—are in fact ways to switch whether Qi is directed inward or outward, which enables the martial artist to convert and release Qi (known as Fajin) or to reserve that energy. Understanding the relation of body structure and Qi flow is absolutely crucial. Generating Qi to be harnessed is a vital component of Martial Arts training, which also includes learning how to activate the channels and amplify the energy for its proper expression through muscular action. The movements are pumps that generate, circulate, and ultimately direct Qi whether inward for storage or outward for force. Rooting the body, aligning the posture properly, and employing Song throughout are not only the foundational cornerstones of martial applications, though. These principles cultivate the energy for applications, but even more importantly, they are the soil of living. As Grandmaster Helen Wu often repeats, people forget that self-defense in the Martial Arts is about survival, and staying alive by being healthy is the greatest form of self-defense.

The body absorbs, generates, emits, and circulates Qi, and that uninterrupted cycle improves overall health. As *The Book of Balance and Energy* states, "Refining energy is a matter of preserving the body" (Cleary 2003b, p.413); or as the Yellow Emperor explains in even greater detail:

> The Yang qi of the body is like the sun. If the sun loses its brilliance or illuminating effect, all things on earth become inactive. The sun is the ultimate Yang. This heavenly energy of the sun, yang qi, surrounds the earth. Correspondingly, in the body this means that the yang qi circulates around the center or core and has the function of protecting the body. (Ni 1995, p.8)

Health, protection, and ultimately life depend on the cultivation, generation, circulation, and refinement of Qi. If Qi is diminished, the body stagnates, and, at its most extreme level of inactivity, the body dies.

Qi is the fuel of life. Quite simply, to maintain the health of the body is to facilitate Qi to continue to be generated and circulated so that life itself continues. But to be alive is not merely to be a body—healthy or not. Living must serve other purposes, which is why Traditional Chinese Medicine emphasizes the interrelationship of Three Treasures—Qi, Jing, and Shen, or energy, vitality, and spirit. The Qi of the body serves the higher purposes of mind and heart, as well as spirit, but if the body is plagued by disease, illness, weakness, fatigue, pain, and other physical ailments, the activities of the mind and heart—and ultimately for Shen (spirit)—are obstructed and the fullness of life is diminished since Qi must be directed to healing and maintaining health. The continued focus on well-being is not the goal, though. The goal is broader in its reach. As one of the ancient maxims states so succinctly, "With your whole being, develop your life." Training the body is life training. The roots of that training move in two directions: inward and deeper into the self, and outward and into the world. Qi is the force that binds heaven and earth to the individual. It entwines the body (Jing/earth) and the spirit (Shen/heaven) and pulses like a river back and forth between the two forging an intimate connection between each individual and the world.

To study and nurture the life of Qi extends beyond the body and branches outward into the ways in which the world impacts the self. As Chapter 1 explains, a range of things impact Qi—from the things that sustain the physical body (food, sleep, air) to things that affect our psychological and emotional state (emotions, stress, work, relationships). The individual decision-making process affects Qi and those decisions establish a foundation for the inherent value and focus of that life. The self is an intricately connected whole. The mind and body are united, and anything that impacts the mind affects the body, and vice versa. The same applies to Qi. As the saying goes: "When the mind is tense, the body is tense. When the body is tense, the Qi is tense."

The life of Qi is a loop connecting body and mind, and tense body Qi returns back to the mind, perpetuating the cycle of tightness, anxiety, fear, unhappiness, pain, and disease, which then returns to affect the condition of body in a self-perpetuating circle. Being physically healthy is a necessary condition to break this cycle of emotional, psychological, and physical "dis-ease." The time-tested strategies of relaxing the body, mind, and heart open the path of health and healing. A classic maxim exclaims that "Song and Jing (tranquility) are the reasons why Qigong can heal you." To reach a state of calm tranquility, a person needs to train diligently in the art of relaxation and continuously monitoring and addressing any impediments that obstruct Song. To achieve a state of perpetual awareness and Song is the goal of many spiritual traditions such as Buddhism and Taoism, which is often rendered as a state of lasting peace and engaged tranquility of being. To be aware, relaxed, and undisturbed is the heart of Song. And the individual must train continuously to be transparent and unruffled in the face of nonstop adversities—the "winds" of circumstance—that life constantly presents.

To be aware of these inevitable winds is not to be fixated upon the negative and "dis-ease" of body, heart, and mind. Rather, awareness is to feel the pulse of Qi that shapes the self and the world. To sense that pulse enables us to respond to it and use it to deepen our perceptions and to create a more intimate and accepting relationship with ourselves and the world. Qi opens ever broadening vistas of the self and beyond, and we can relax feeling its currents move through our bodies as it does through all things.

CHAPTER 4

Powered by Breath

The silver door slid open and unfamiliar faces stared out as I stepped into the elevator. I reached over to push the button for the twenty-third floor of the headquarters of a large health insurance company. Everyone was dressed in corporate business attire, but I was wearing loose workout pants and a t-shirt with the logo of my studio, Still Mountain T'ai Chi and Chi Kung, since I was heading to the weekly Taiji and Qigong seminar that I teach for doctors and executives. Already feeling out of place, I could feel someone's intent gaze upon me. Then a voice broke the silence and I realized the question was directed to me: "Why are you powered by air?" I swiveled my head around somewhat perplexed and said "Excuse me?" And the man then added, "Your shirt, it says you are powered by air." A few people shuffled uncomfortably and someone chortled. Then I put it together. I was wearing my studio shirt with "Powered by Qi" on the back. The Chinese character for Qi is in the center of a circle that has "Powered By" on the top and "Still Mountain" on the bottom. I replied to the man, "That character is Qi or energy, which includes air. The shirt is supposed to be a joke." The humor missed the mark with the elevator crowd, and uncomfortable silence enveloped the space again. When the elevator reached the twenty-third floor, I was the only one who stepped off, and as the doors closed, I let all of the awkwardness dissolve into a quiet laugh.

Of course, the man's interpretation of the Chinese calligraphy and his question weren't wrong. The character for Qi is composed of two parts—"air" and "uncooked rice" (food). Air and breath are so vital to Qi that some people even translate the word "Qigong" as "breath work" and focus exclusively on holding specific postures and using the breath to circulate Qi. There is a rich tradition of such techniques called Wai Dan (External Elixir) and Nei Dan (Internal Elixir), the history of which stretches back thousands of years. A set attributed to the Ch'an Buddhist patriarch, Bodhidharma, is one of the most famous, during which stationary postures are held to build energy in the Dantian and direct Qi to specific parts of the body. The first posture of the set will be described later in this chapter as a way to show how the breath, body, and Qi come together in the practice. Suffice it to say for now that the breath techniques amplify the generation and accelerate the building up of Qi; or to put it more poetically, breath fans the fire of Qi.

Many ancient Taoist sources refer to the breath as the "bellows" because of its ability to increase Qi in the body by working in coordination with the "furnace" (body and Dantian) to fire the "cauldron" (the mind and spiritual pursuits). The respiratory process fuels the Qi in the body which can be led to the mind for spiritual practices. The breath is the bridge between the physical body and the mind, and links the perceptible, physical workings of the body and the invisible, abstract processes of the mind: the breath is physical (it fills and expands the lungs and can be felt) and yet abstract (it is invisible). Perhaps it is that dual nature as perceptible and yet ephemeral that gives breath its connection to spiritual traditions and the sacred: the breath of the Divine, for example, the focal point of meditative practices, or the Christian sense of God breathing life into the first human, Adam. As *Taoist Meditation*, a classic Taoist sourcebook, puts it so elegantly, "Human energy is always in communion with heaven and earth in the alteration of exhalation and inhalation" (Cleary 2000, p.11). The breath moves back and forth between heaven and earth, Yin and Yang. Lao Tzu describes such movement as well:

> *The space between heaven and earth*
> *is like bellows and pipes,*
> *empty yet inexhaustible,*
> *producing more with movement.*
>
> (CLEARY 1992, P.11)

Breath sparks life and powers all living things. Breath is a vital tool of living that exists at the threshold of heaven and earth, and when used properly it has the potential to open the threshold onto the sacred. Movement—of the body, the breath, and the mind—also produces more: more energy, more vitality, more spirit.

The physical, energetic, and spiritual cannot be divorced from one another any more than body, breath, and mind are separate aspects of a sentient being. The breath feeds the body and mind just as Qi fuels Shen and Jing, which creates a whole. Nevertheless, to explore Qi in greater depth moves from the substance of the body and toward the mind, and the intermediary that bridges the two is the breath. In the language of Taoist sources, the breath fans the flames of the furnace, and that energy can be used to forge the mind and expand the self. How breath works in coordination with the body to generate Qi, and how the breath is inextricably intertwined with spiritual cultivation of tranquility and Shen, is the open secret of breath's latent power—the power to fuel life.

Regulating Body, Breath, and Mind

Classic training in the Internal Martial Arts proposes that there are five areas of concentration, each of which is related to and enhances the others. These are what are known as the five regulations, or training body, breath, mind, Qi, and spirit.[13] The first three areas correspond to the furnace (body), bellows (breath) and cauldron (mind)—all of which generate, regulate, and direct the Qi. The last two areas of regulating Qi and spirit (Shen) build upon the foundation of the body, breath, and mind and turn the focus to harnessing that energy for regulating health and wellness as well as transforming Qi for spiritual cultivation. Each of these areas overlaps with the others, so it would be remiss, if not impossible, to discuss them as independent areas of training. A tense body obstructs breathing, for example, which agitates the mind and impedes the flow of Qi. Proper training means being aware of the body, breath, and mind working together, and the act of regulating means paying attention to all three. Traditional Chinese Medicine regards the body as an interrelated whole as well, and to treat a specific problem (a skin rash, for example) requires not just treating the site of the problem (the skin), but the organs and channels as well (the lungs, in this case). The body's organs, channels, and the mind, and all of their processes, are one unit too: the respiratory process is the manifestation of the state of the body and mind; the emotional and psychological state of the mind is affected by the condition of the body; and the mind impacts the state of the body. Just as a tense body creates tense Qi, when the breath is shallow and tight, the Qi is weak and constricted.

The relationship between body and breath can be demonstrated quite easily by raising the shoulders and feeling how the breath concentrates into the upper chest and respiration becomes more shallow and rapid. When the shoulders are relaxed and lowered, the sternum hollows, and the breath is able to reach deeper, past the diaphragm and into the lower portion of the lungs, which allows the breath to soften and become fuller. Yang Cheng Fu's explanation of the impact of the tightness of the shoulders upon the power of the body (discussed in the previous chapter) applies to the quality of breath as well. Yang explains that "If you cannot relax and sink, the two shoulders will be raised up and tense. The Qi will follow them and the whole body cannot get power." The breath follows tense shoulders upward, and the inability to relax and sink alters the breath and adds to the drain of power. While the body needs to be relaxed, properly structured, and centered in order to cultivate Qi, the breath also needs to be unobstructed and full in order to build Qi; when it is not full, the respiratory process contributes to the depletion of power. Just as the state of relaxation allows an individual to feel the body more deeply, Song facilitates deeper breathing and the ability to tap the full potential of the lungs to power the body.

Traditional Chinese Medicine conceptualizes the lungs as having four sections: the front, back, right side, and left side, which can be divided into upper and lower quadrants as well. While the lungs really only have two physical lobes, organs in Traditional Chinese Medicine are defined not by physical form but by process. The Triple Heater, an important organ in Chinese Medicine, loosely corresponds to the three sections of the torso—the upper, middle, and lower heaters, or "burners"—which regulate the circulation and energy in those three respective areas that include the Liver, Spleen, Kidney, Heart, and Lung. Yet there isn't an identifiable Triple Heater organ for each burner, but rather a region of the body where the process takes place. Similarly, the lungs consist of four interrelated sections. The strongest part of the lungs tends to be the upper front since most people favor this area, which is also why a person when "winded" by physical exertion will often bend forward at the waist and place the hands on the thighs or knees: the upper front of the lungs are tired from the exertion, and the bending forward directs air into the back of the lungs, which have not been overextended and remain "fresher."

Leaning forward to breathe into the back exemplifies how the position of the body impacts which part of the lungs is engaged during respiration. Bending, stretching, and physical posture makes it possible to "aim" the breath into a section of the lungs. Raised shoulders, for example, forces the breath into the upper front and back of the lungs; relaxed shoulders also relaxes the center of the sternum, which allows the breath to reach into the lower lungs; and the sides of the lungs can be engaged by stretching the sides and rotating the waist. To breathe to these different portions of the lungs stimulates the blood into those areas as well. Since Qi is the force behind the blood (called nutritive Qi or Ying qi), respiratory technique helps to deliver blood and Qi throughout the capillary system of the entire lungs. Not coincidentally, many forms of lung cancer and bacterial infections begin in the outer reaches of the lungs, since the upper lungs are often favored and the lower portions are used less, meaning that blood flow is decreased in those areas. Furthermore, stress and anxiety add to physical tension, which further constricts air flow and impedes breathing into the lower and side areas of the lungs. Shallow breathing creates fertile soil for an illness to take hold in the lungs. The overall health of the body is a direct result of the quality and character of respiration. Fully engaging all parts of the lungs maintains the entire Qi system since respiratory process is the bellows for the body—pumping Qi and blood through the channels. Proper breathing is a cornerstone of overall health and well-being.

Deep Long Slow Soft Even Tranquil

The qualities of proper breathing adhere to six attributes. The physical qualities are that the breath is *deep*, *long*, *slow*, and *soft*; and the two other—*even* and *tranquil*—are by-products of these physical characteristics. All of these qualities lead into the others, but one might visualize this breath like a stream of air passing through a slim tube from the nose and into the lower abdomen. The thin stream reaches deeply into the body by following a slow, steady pathway. For the breath to be long, air cannot be "gulped" through the mouth; instead, inhalation and exhalation is through the nose, which keeps the breath soft. A deep, long, slow, and soft breath allows the inhalation and exhalation to be even, creating a smooth respiratory cycle. Collectively, these qualities generate an overall feeling of physical and mental tranquility. To breathe deep, long, slow, and soft engages all four quadrants of the lungs, which not only takes pressure off of the heart and lungs, but also makes the pumping of Qi throughout the body more efficient and smooth. The ability to direct Qi with the breath builds upon these six qualities.

The previous chapter (Chapter 3) analyzes how physical movement can direct Qi to a specific part of the body, to an organ, and/or channels of the body, and when coupled with physical action, the process of inhalation and exhalation creates an internal massage that stimulates circulation further. The lungs, too, can be targeted by using different breathing techniques that direct Qi into specific areas of the lungs themselves while simultaneously concentrating Qi in differing parts of the body. The internal massage of an organ or a channel is a product of the act of respiration wherein the diaphragmatic and muscular movement creates and releases pressure that stimulates the circulation and drives the Qi. There are three rudimentary breathing styles that circulate and propel Qi, each of which is performed differently and, as a result, has diverse effects on Qi. The first style is Chest, which is often a natural response to stress and anxiety, but can used for strenuous activities such as lifting weights or the external Martial Arts exercise of breaking boards, bricks, and other objects. The other two techniques, which are central to the Internal Arts of Taiji, Qigong, and meditation, are Abdominal Breathing and Reverse Abdominal Breathing. Abdominal Breathing is also known as "Buddhist Breathing" since it is linked to Ch'an meditative practices, and Reverse Abdominal Breathing is often called "Taoist Breathing" since it is fundamental to the Taoist technique of transforming Qi into Shen.

Numerous mainstream health publications as well as peer-reviewed medical studies agree that chest breathing is by far the predominant way in which most people breath. To chest breathe, an individual expands the chest and/or lifts the shoulders, which concentrates the breath into the upper quadrant. This kind of breathing is a natural response to fight-or-flight stimuli, which generates energy for quick action, but it also creates tightness in the chest and back. The Traditional Chinese Medicine principle of how a muscular action in coordination with respiration creates internal organ pressure explains how chest breathing pushes upon the heart, causing the pace to quicken, and accelerates blood circulation into the large muscles. This response is a natural reaction to perceived dangers and stressful situations, and directs Qi outward into the skin and muscles for immediate action. The flowing of blood and Qi into the muscles is accompanied by a draining of blood from the extremities including the brain. When a person is frightened, the common saying is that he or she turns "white as a sheet" since the blood drains from the face and is redirected into the quadriceps, pectoral muscles, deltoids, and biceps.

The flow of the blood and Qi into muscles is the reason behind the fact that the same breath is used to lift or move a heavy object. The quick, sharp inhalation pressurizes the heart, and blood courses into the muscles. Chest breathing is a natural response to certain situations, but continuous chest breathing perpetuates a physical tightness in the body as well as a feeling of stress, both of which use excessive energy. While this breathing technique is task specific, continuous chest breathing has a negative cumulative effect on health since it perpetuates the conditions and causes of stress and heightened anxiety. A number of the published studies on breathing claim that over 80 percent of people breathe only with the chest, which may point to, or be the product of, the modern epidemic of stress, anxiety, and cardiopulmonary disease. Many of these same studies suggest that Abdominal Breathing is the most appropriate remedy; or as we probably have been told at some point in our life: take a deep breath.

Breathe Like a Buddhist/Breathe Like a Taoist

The documented health benefits of Abdominal Breathing include such things as alleviating stress, reducing and helping to manage anxiety, lowering blood pressure, managing pain, and generating a sense of relaxation and well-being. A wide range of sources from medical studies to articles and books published for a mainstream audience recommend Abdominal Breathing as the most ideal way to maintain health and well-being.[14] The basic gist of Abdominal Breathing is that as a person inhales, the diaphragm extends downward, which allows the lungs to drop into the abdominal cavity. Buddhist breathing adds a further ripple beyond just breathing deeply: as the diaphragm drops, the area between the anus and the genitals, known as the Huiyin, presses downward, and the abdominal wall, the lower back, and Mingmen press outward. The abdomen, lower back, Huiyin, and diaphragm return to a neutral or natural starting position with the exhalation. The Buddhist technique of inhalation and exhalation is coordinated with muscular movement as shown in Figure 4.1.

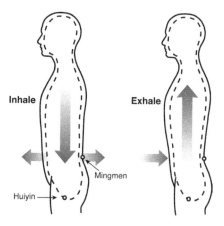

FIGURE 4.1 ABDOMINAL OR BUDDHIST BREATHING

As the breath is directed downward, the lower abdomen expands much the same as a baby's belly inflates like a balloon while breathing, which is why this technique is sometimes referred to as "Baby Breathing." One of the hypotheses explaining why babies breathe in this manner is that this muscular abdominal contraction draws nutrients from the mother through the umbilical cord like a pump. While this theory cannot be verified, it suggests an intriguing correlation wherein the physical movement facilitates the sharing of prenatal jing and nutritive Qi. Regardless of whether or not Abdominal Breathing was for absorbing Qi while in the womb, Buddhist Breathing is an invaluable means for circulating Qi throughout the body, as well as increasing the flow to the internal organs and especially to the Kidney, which helps to store energy in the Dantian.

Reverse Abdominal Breathing pumps Qi as well, but it is performed with one significant difference: during Abdominal Breathing the gates of the diaphragm and Huiyin press downward with inhalation; Reversal Abdominal Breathing constricts the diaphragm and Huiyin inward and upward during inhalation. The constriction of the diaphragm causes it to flatten and broaden, expanding the ribs outward. Pressure is exerted from the diaphragm and Huiyin— constricting the front and lower abdominal walls that press upon the Dantian. Like the Abdominal Breathing, though, the lower back and Mingmen expand outward with inhalation. During exhalation, each of these areas of the body release and return to the neutral or natural starting position, which is shown in Figure 4.2.

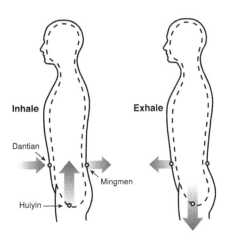

FIGURE 4.2 REVERSE ABDOMINAL OR TAOIST BREATHING

Reverse Abdominal or Taoist Breathing circulates Qi to the internal organs, but greater amounts of Qi are directed into the extremities such as the hands and head. To draw Qi into the upper Dantian, located in the cerebral cortex of the brain, is a core method in Taoist Meditation and body practices where the energy is intended to be led into the mind and transformed into Shen or spiritual consciousness.

Proper Abdominal Breathing and Reverse Abdominal Breathing builds upon the fundamental body principles covered in Chapter 3: the body must be relaxed and adhere to the principle of Song; proper structure, stance, and rootedness help to facilitate proper breathing; and the body should be centered. These principles open the gates of the body so that the breath can adhere to qualities of being *deep*, *long*, *slow*, and *soft*—*even* and creating *tranquility*. In this state, breath aids in the circulation of Qi through the Small Circuit or Microcosmic Orbit (see Figure 4.3). In addition to these body principles, the tongue rests behind the top front teeth on what is called the heart palate, which reinforces respiration through the nose while also connecting the circuit of the Microcosmic Orbit (the Governing Channel that runs from the Dantian down to Huiyin, then up the back, over the crown of the head and Baihui, and finishing beneath the nose; and the Conception Channel, which goes from beneath the lower lip and runs down the front of the body to the Dantian). The breathing cycle helps to guide Qi through the entire circuit, as shown in Figure 4.3.

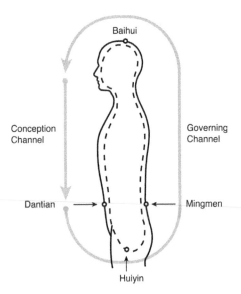

FIGURE 4.3 THE SMALL CIRCUIT OR MICROCOSMIC ORBIT

Using either the Buddhist or Taoist method, the breath can be used to guide and feel the Qi moving through the body. There are a diverse range of variants for how to perform Small Circulation (or Microcosmic) Breathing. Described here is one version that is both simple and effective. To practice the Microcosmic or Small Circulation training, first breathe in and out naturally and deeply using either the Buddhist or Taoist technique. Once the connection between body, breath, mind, and Qi is made, begin with an inhalation into the abdomen and lead Qi from the Dantian through Huiyin and Mingmen and up the back to the base of the neck, which is called the Jade Pillow or Da Zhui (located at C7, the large vertebra at the intersection of the neck and shoulders), continuing to Baihui at the crown of the head and finishing underneath the nose. Exhale and lead the breath down the front of the body back to the Dantian. If blockages along the path obstruct feeling the breath, multiple breath cycles can be used to help build Qi and direct the breath. Once this becomes smooth, one breath cycle is ideal since the breath cycle operates similar to barometric pressure. Breathing into the abdomen increases the compression on the Dantian, which then propels Qi through the main Governing and Conception channels, and, in turn, into the other channels, which branch out from the Governing and Conception channels. The breath strengthens the stream of Qi flowing through the body.

The relaxed stance opens the lungs and the respiratory pathways so that the breath can sink into the lower abdomen without any physical obstructions and reach the Dantian. Muscular movement at the Dantian creates a pump that circulates blood and Qi. But Buddhist and Taoist techniques lead the Qi to different sites in the body. The Buddhist approach of expanding the belly with the inhalation extends the Dantian, Mingmen, and Huiyin outward, and the returning to a neutral position with the exhalation generates a gentle inward pressure which stimulates Qi circulation. Since the physical action expands at the Dantian and Mingmen, the Governing and Conception channels are engaged and activate Qi through the Microcosmic Orbit. Buddhist breathing fills the Dantian, which is often referred to as a vessel or reservoir for Qi, and then circulates Qi to the internal organs and to the channels of the limbs with the exhalation. Pressure is alleviated from the heart as well, allowing the heart rate to decrease even as the oxygenation of the body is increased. Serotonin, a mood-stabilizing neurotransmitter, is also released, which deepens the state of physical and mental relaxation while simultaneously increasing the feeling of being awake and alert. Whereas the chest breathing perpetuates a self-sustaining cycle of tension and anxiety, Abdominal Breathing prompts the body, heart, and mind to be more at ease.

Reverse Abdominal Breathing or Taoist Breathing generates an internal pressure upon the Dantian with the inhalation, and as the breath draws in, the diaphragm is flattened—pressing outward and expanding the sides of the lungs. The abdominal muscles and the lungs are engaged, creating an inward pressure upon the Dantian that drives Qi through the Microcosmic Orbit. Reverse Abdominal creates a pocket of internal compression with the inhalation that is released with the exhalation, and the "massaging" of the Dantian is much more direct than the Abdominal Breathing technique, and generates a much more invigorating and less relaxing feeling than the Buddhist Breathing method.

An appropriate analogy for these two styles might be that Buddhist Breathing is like a cup of green tea: relaxing with a steady warming of the body. Taoist Breathing is an espresso: invigorating, uplifting, and stimulating. The effects and benefits differ slightly between the two. The key benefits of Abdominal/Buddhist Breathing include:

- internal organ massage

- invigoration of abdominal muscles

- increase of Qi to the Kidney, and directing of Qi to the Dantian and storage there

- increase of what is called water Qi, which calms the mind, strengthens the Will, and firms the Shen (spirit).

The increase in water Qi is crucial for moving and seated Ch'an Buddhism, wherein the energy is used to fuel the awareness and concentration of extended meditative sessions. The cumulative effect of calmness and awareness is used to awaken Buddha nature—the inherent mind that is unencumbered by the attachments and desires that do not allow a person to be fully present and at one with the flow of the Tao.

The benefits of Taoist Breathing, on the other hand, include:

- Qi is led to the internal organs.

- Greater amounts of Qi are directed into the extremities of the body.

- It generates Jin—the force and the Will of Martial Arts.

- It increases guardian Qi (called Wei Qi), which protects the body from illness.

- It raises Qi for bone marrow washing and other techniques used for Iron Body training.

Taoist Breathing increases Qi to the surface areas of the body, which is one of the reasons why many hard-style Qigong practices utilize this technique in Iron Body training where one part of the body is strengthened by concentrating Qi to that area. Taoist Breathing technique is an extremely fast way of generating Qi wherein each breath and muscular contraction stimulates the Dantian by filling and compressing. This technique also expedites Qi to the Five Gates of the palms, feet, and crown of the head, which sends Qi outward. Reverse Abdominal Breathing generates a steady supply of Qi to the organs and channels, but more energy is focused outward, and the Taoist approach should be used in conjunction with exercises that store and harmonize the body's energy so that health is not compromised through the loss of excessive Qi. Many Qigong sets, for example, incorporate "recovery moves" as a way to harmonize and balance the body by releasing surplus Qi and simultaneously storing essential energy to preserve health and longevity.

Breathe with Body

Buddhist and Taoist Breath methods are tools to generate and direct the flow of Qi either inward or outward, and are used in coordination with specific muscular movement. Yet the flow of Qi happens naturally and without conscious effort, which can be demonstrated in a simple exercise where body and breath are naturally synchronized. Pick an object and continuously gaze at it. Breathing naturally, feel how the eyes widen with the inhalation as if the breath "takes in" the view. Now reverse the process. Open the eyes wider with the exhalation, which will feel unnatural, forced, and awkward. The eyes open and pupils dilate in conjunction with the inhalation in order to absorb light, which is a form of Qi. The breath and body seamlessly work together, and while certain techniques can be utilized to increase and focus that energy, the process happens naturally and without conscious effort with each respiratory cycle. The eyes, mouth, and nose are gates where Qi enters and exits, and respiration functions like a valve directing the flow inward or outward.

Another example of how the body and breath seamlessly and naturally function in respect to Qi is discussed in the previous chapter (Chapter 3), in which the technique of gently holding the breath while pulling the abdominal muscles inward is used as a way to help feel and locate the Dantian. This technique requires a small amount of conscious engagement in order to perform the muscular contraction and holding of the breath, but the mind isn't explicitly "leading" the Qi; rather, the mind is paying attention to the feeling of Qi being generated in the Dantian. In that exercise too the breath is used to direct the Qi inward, and gently holding the breath closes the valve and pressurizes the Qi within the Dantian, which is amplified through the slight muscular constriction. What is felt isn't so much the Dantian, but the accumulation of Qi *within* the Dantian: the compression of the abdominal cavity builds Qi. Subsequently, the Dantian is sometimes translated as "Energy Seed Field" which seems highly appropriate since the drawing of light in through the eyes and the stimulation from the breath are sparks that enable Qi to grow. While Qi naturally occurs in the body, the Dantian is the soil that can be nurtured and tended through body techniques and respiratory methods—thereby transforming that soil into a "field" of Qi.

These two examples demonstrate that the body and breath naturally and unconsciously work together in sustaining and processing Qi. The methods of Buddhist, Taoist, and Microcosmic Breathing build upon this natural foundation in order to amplify and harness that Qi to increase circulation for the purposes of health, well-being, and spiritual pursuits. Being able to feel the connections between body, breath, and Qi is a necessary step in being able to lead Qi; or to put it in different terms, recognizing and feeling the alteration of exhalation and inhalation is to be in the flow of Yin and Yang, which the ancient Taoist sources tell us is to be in "communion with heaven and earth."

The Language of Tiger and Dragon Qi

Terms such as "Energy Seed Field" and "Mud Pill Palace" and instructions to "Breathe to the Heels" and even being "in communion with heaven and earth" seem to be coded language that obscures or hides the real meaning. Such language, unfortunately, has led to a great deal of misinterpretation and errors leading practitioners further astray from the essence of Qi. The seemingly veiled language is not intended to hide the "secrets" of Qi but to point to the essence and *feeling* of the practice. Such language is supposed to help, not hinder, by demonstrating *how* the methods might feel when done correctly. Neither those "feelings" nor the outcomes of the techniques are intended to be prescriptive or the "goal" of practice, but rather an attempt to spark an individual's own personal discovery of the life of Qi. After all, what does an "Energy Seed" feel like? The term is a pointer—a metaphor that alludes to the outline of the experience. It is not the full disclosure of the experience, nor is it the indication that the person has now gotten "it." Examples abound in Taoist and Buddhist sources and Martial Arts training manuals of such pointers, but one is particularly relevant to breath and Qi—namely, phrases about breathing like a tiger and/or a dragon. While the characters of the tiger and the dragon may seem very similar, these two present different flavors of Qi. Tiger breath is Yin and Dragon breath is Yang, which may seem perplexing since they both seem like "Yang" creatures. Beyond these superficial parallels, the distinctive and differing qualities of the tiger and dragon provide a nuanced view of how Qi can be utilized for different ends—either through directing the breath and Qi inward or outward.

Inhalation is Yin—gathering and drawing inward—which is associated with the tiger. That the tiger is Yin may seem odd since it is a ferocious hunter. What makes it such a tremendous predator is its constant awareness (eyes open and alert) coupled with its ability to remain still and camouflaged. The energy of the tiger is like a coiled spring poised to act. The tiger remains vigilant, accumulating energy that is stored but ever prepared to spring into action. The relationship of awareness and gathering of potential energy is implicit in the Five Animals Qigong for Tiger wherein the movements target the liver (which stores and processes blood) and the eyes (the windows of awareness). In Traditional Chinese Medicine the eyes and liver are connected. All of these connotations surrounding the tiger continue to point to various ways in which the pathway of Qi is absorbed inward through the eyes, blood, and breath. To breathe like a tiger is the Yin act of gathering energy and is used to be tigerlike: alert and aware, with stores of latent energy. The earlier exercise in which the eyes naturally widen with inhalation is being like a tiger. The character of the inhalation is to take in, be alert and aware, and store energy for use. The tiger breath has a purpose beyond being merely an unconscious activity and requires vigilant concentration. As such, to breathe like a tiger is to draw in with all of the senses.

The dragon, on the other hand, is usually depicted in Chinese painting and other iconography as soaring, swimming, in a whirlwind of smoke, water, clouds, fire, and energy. Dragon is the ultimate representative of Yang:

dynamic, active, moving, and fierce. Even its breath emerges from its mouth and nostrils in a swirl of smoke and heat. Qi is released with the breath as well through exhalation through the mouth and nose. Exhaling through the mouth propels Qi outward, and one of the classic sounds that martial artists employ is "ha" to accompany a particularly dynamic move or application. The execution of the sound increases the force of the movement, thereby using the focused breath to strengthen the physical action. Similarly, in Six Sacred Syllable Qigong, the practitioner uses "he" to release heart and its channels. The exhalation coupled with the vocalization not only affects specific organs and channels by sound vibrations but also emits energy. Qi is emitted through the air and vocalization through the mouth during talking, for example, which helps to explain why long conversations often leave the participants feeling tired. Too much Qi is dispersed with too much talking! This may also explain why silence is standard monastic protocol since one is preserving Qi for sacred practices. To breathe like a dragon propels the Qi outward and generates force or Jin, which can explode like a dragon's breath in a dynamic cloud of heat and energy. Exhalation leads the Qi outward, although closing the mouth and exhaling through the nose retains more energy. As the breath exits the body, Qi streams into the arm and leg channels as well as to the Five Gates of the palms, head, and balls of the feet. To use the breath to guide Qi in this way is what is known as Classic Gate Breathing, a simple and effective exercise that demonstrates how Qi is released naturally with a Yang dragon breath.

Feeling and Focusing Breath and Qi

To properly execute Gate Breathing, the body needs to be in a state of relaxation and in proper alignment and stance, then raise both hands to the sides of the face with the palms facing inward. Begin by using the Taoist/Reverse Abdominal Breathing technique with the inhalations and exhalations following the qualities of deep, long, slow, and soft. Concentrate the attention on the space between the palms and the face. A natural pause between inhalation and exhalation should occur, and gradually heat will increase with each exhalation and during the pause prior to inhaling again. Then try the same technique, but with the exhalation, breathe out through the mouth. Then repeat the same thing again but vocalize "he" with the exhalation. The intensity of the heat between face and palms changes with the alteration of the breath. Finally, perform the same exercise but using the Buddhist/Abdominal Breathing technique. Each of these variants produces a different quality and intensity of energy.

This basic principle of using breath to generate and lead Qi is the foundation of many Internal Arts practices. One of the most profound Qigong sets, Wai Dan, guides energy simply with breath and mind. In the basic stationary forms of Wai Dan, a posture is held and the practitioner visualizes engaging the muscles in a particular way while coordinating respiration to match the move. For example, in the first posture, stand with the feet shoulder width and the body relaxed and aligned (Figure 4.4). The elbows are slightly bent with both hands at the sides with the palms held parallel to the ground and the fingers pointing forward.

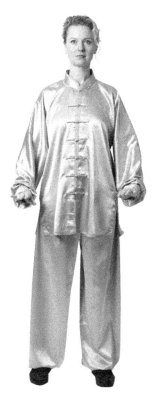

FIGURE 4.4 WAI DAN QIGONG FIRST POSTURE

Inhale a deep natural breath using Buddhist technique, and with the exhalation imagine pushing the palms downward and pulling the fingers upward. The hands do not move, but the action is imagined, which activates the muscular and energetic channels. The person then visualizes releasing and relaxing the muscles with the exhalation. The combination of mind, breath, and body activates the Yang channels (outside) of the arms and directs Qi into the wrists, hands, and fingers. In this particular stationary Qigong form, which includes twelve total postures, the energy builds in different parts of the body, and in the first stance, Qi builds in the wrists. The same principle of building Qi is behind Sun Lu Tang's modification of the San Ti posture with the wrists bent and fingers pointing upward in order to generate, concentrate, and retain the Qi of the body. When the wrist is straightened and the fingers point forward, the Qi is dispersed.

Furnace, Bellows, Cauldron

Wai Dan Qigong illustrates how body, breath, and mind are integrated in the cultivation and use of Qi, and together these three things comprise the total, interrelated energy system of the body, with each part being necessary and vital. At the same time, each performs a separate task and has a somewhat unique role. The body is the fundamental framework—the furnace—within which Qi is accumulated, generated, concentrated, and stored. The mind, which is sometimes referred to as the General or Emperor, directs and controls the body, breath, and energetic system. The mind, though, depends on the body and breath to provide the energetic sustenance for the mind to continue leading. Breath is the intermediary between body and mind, and provides the power to increase the Qi of the body which can be used by the mind. The respiratory process harnesses the power of air in order to activate and increase the energy that streams between body and mind, heaven and earth. In this way, breath is the fuel for keeping the body and mind healthy, and our breathing is the sign of the quality of our being—whether relaxed or tense, active or stagnant. And it is a tool to make changes that improve our health, well-being, and quality of life.

If we want an accurate understanding of the state of the body and mind, the breath yields immediate insights. As the ancestral Taoist teacher Qui is quoted as saying in *Taoist Meditation*, "If the breathing is at all unsettled, life is not your own" (Cleary 2000, p.23). The state of the breath— short, shallow, labored—reveals the condition of the body and mind—tight, ill, in pain, distressed, anxious— and when the body and mind are in a state of "dis-ease," it is very difficult to be present, aware, and to be able to devote oneself to purposes other than dealing with pain and discomfort of the present situation. "When the breath is settled," that famous Taoist Ancestor Liu tells us, "the spirit settles with it. This is what is referred to as real people breathing from their heels" (Cleary 2000, p.25). Mastering the breath is key to becoming a "real" person," which is the Taoist way of saying that a person has become enlightened and is now a complete human being fully integrated with the Tao.

While the goal of becoming an "enlightened" being may seem beyond our reach, being a more balanced, healthy, and contented person *is* within our power. To learn how to settle the breath is not only the pathway to health and well-being, it opens the practitioner to the ability to harness the power of spirit. Breath is the "real bellows" that fans the furnace of the body, and that combined energy is directed to the cauldron—the mind—which houses consciousness and being. Breath is life, but the contours and shape of that life depend on how a person uses the body's raw material energy and cultivates the tools of the bellows to shape and refine that material. The real power of breath is that it can be used to forge a real life out of Qi—a life that is healthy, vital, and full of purpose.

CHAPTER 5

Cultivating Mind and Heart

The hands on the clock crept closer and closer to 9:00 a.m., and with each passing minute, my pacing back and forth to the parking lot grew in intensity. I shuffled nervously from the large room that held nearly fifty people to the entranceway to peer out hoping to see my friend, mentor, and coach, Grandmaster Nick Gracenin, whom I had invited to offer the very first workshop in my T'ai Chi and Internal Arts Institute. I was already anxious since this was the first time I was moving ahead with my plan to bring gifted teachers and recognized Internal Artist masters to Pittsburgh to share their expertise. Grandmaster Gracenin was driving in to teach a daylong session on Baguazhang, the swirling dynamic Internal Martial Art. As the inaugural workshop for the new program, I was very apprehensive that the sessions would be successful enough to continue, and the clock creeping closer to the start time with the key teacher yet to arrive didn't seem to bode well for the future.

With minutes to spare, a car pulled into the parking lot, and Grandmaster Gracenin hopped out, lifted his sunglasses, and calmly greeted me: "Hi. Great to see you. I was stuck in detour traffic." His matter-of-fact calmness was offset by my polite but nervous attempt to steer him into the room to start the workshop. Completely nonplussed and right on time, he walked into the room and patiently began to unpack his bag as fifty faces turned to study him. When he had emptied the bag of books, DVDs, shoes, and other materials, he said:

> Good Morning. I am glad to be here, but I had some difficulty because of road construction. Every detour seemed to take me farther from where I needed to be, and at one point I had no idea where I was. But then I thought, *how appropriate that I am going to teach Bagua since Bagua is all about change and learning to move with that change.* And here I am. Let's begin.

With that introduction, the art of Bagua was transformed into a life lesson and the essence of the art was modeled perfectly for the participants: to accept and move with change is to adapt to the necessary detours, not be subsumed by the frustration of the situation, and remain calmly in the present. On the other hand, despite my decades of meditation and Internal Arts training, not to mention the years of teaching people how to relax, I was anxious. Nervous. Distracted. And I had even forgotten my favorite saying: "Everything always works out one way or the other." And it did work out. Grandmaster Gracenin had arrived in time, the session was brilliant, and it was indeed a sign for the future success of the T'ai Chi and Internal Arts Institute, which has been humming along for many years now.

I learned a great deal that day about the real lessons of the Internal Arts and the mind.

The Power of Change

While the health of the body sustains us, and without which we cannot exist, and the breath provides the sustenance to power the body, it is the mind that is ultimately the key to providing value, purpose, and reason for life. And it is the mind that has the greatest potential to wreck havoc on the health of the body and dissipate the total fabric of life—the social, work, familial, personal, and spiritual. The mind is the centerpiece in the life of Qi, and it can contribute in a positive or negative way to the entire texture of our being. The ability to change is to recognize and honor the flow of Qi, and that transformation happens in the core of the mind.

Change can be unsettling, and often it throws us for a loop when the plan that we constructed in our heads doesn't match reality. It is the ability to accept and move with change that reveals so much about the latent potentiality of the mind and its ability to float on the stream of life's Qi. The capability to shift perspective and transform an event or happening and ourselves is a natural extension of cultivating and refining energy in such a way that we are transformed into the person that the Yellow Emperor admires:

The sages lived peacefully under heaven on earth, following the rhythms of the planet and the universe. They adapted to society without being swayed by cultural trends. They were free from emotional extremes and lived a balanced, contented existence. Their outward appearance, behavior, and thinking did not reflect the conflicting norms of society. The sages appeared busy but were never depleted. Internally they did not overburden themselves. They abided in calmness, recognizing the empty nature of phenomenological existence. The sages lived over one hundred years because they did not scatter and disperse their energies. (Ni 1995, pp.39–40)

An abundance of energy and an abiding calmness is the outward manifestation of mind, yet to train the mind and use it to cultivate the life of Qi is extremely arduous. Dr. Jwing-Ming Yang once remarked that in respect to the five regulations of classic training, most people can regulate body, many can learn how to regulate breath, but few are able to reach the point where mind is regulated.[15]

What is it that makes training the mind so difficult? Answers to that question stretch back thousands of years, and the core issue has much to do with human nature and the way that attention is distracted and darts from one thing to another in the search for satisfaction and validation. The mind leads the quest for physical, emotional, and psychological fulfillment, but without a deeper understanding, gratification remains perpetually elusive.

Training requires the development of concentration and focus, which harnesses the mind and cultivates calmness and tranquility. Once awareness is sufficiently developed, the mind is capable of regulating Qi and transforming Qi into Shen. The relationship of concentration, mind, and Qi is a self-perpetuating loop: deeper concentration means stronger Yi, and stronger Yi means that Qi flow will be stronger. Building concentration is key; therefore, training requires taming the propensity for distraction—or what the Ancients called the Monkey Mind.

Monkey Mind

The human mind has a tendency to flit from stimulation to stimulation. Contemporary culture sometimes refers to this behavior at its most extreme as attention deficient disorder or hyperactivity. Thousands of years ago it was called Monkey Mind since attention and concentration would leap from thing to thing like a monkey springing from one branch of a tree to another. The analogy is apt since "springing" consumes energy, and just as focus is diffused by the distraction from object to object, so is the mental energy dispersed.

Scattered and quickly shifting attention has its roots in innate survival instincts. To stay out of danger, constant attention to the environment was required and every sensory perception should be observed since it could be a sign of a predator. But as human beings shifted to develop social structures for protection and safety, the habit of rapidly shifting focus remained. While we may not have to worry about predators, our level of distraction remains high. Compounded by this tendency to be distracted are human emotions, concepts of self-image and worth, as well as other manifestations of personal identity. In effect, the mind can be a tangled mess—a veritable jungle of emotional, irrational, and sometimes selfish monkeys. The response to this issue was to develop meditative techniques that strengthen mental focus and nurture self-awareness. Buddhist Meditation, for example, emphasizes that for the mind to be properly cultivated, a practitioner must maintain effort (sustain the energy and Will of training), be mindful (become aware of the self and the world), and develop concentration (focus and direction of attention). Training the mind, in this respect, is akin to using particular exercises to strengthen specific muscles, or repeating certain exercises to refine a set of skills. Meditation strengthens and refines concentrated awareness. Taoism, too, emphasizes the importance of meditation as the cornerstone of spiritual cultivation, and this also applies to the Internal Arts—so much so that Taiji is sometimes referred to as "Moving Meditation."

A classic saying is "One should look inward three times a day." "Looking Inward" is another name for meditative practices, which serve two purposes: first, meditation strengthens concentration and focus; second, that focus enhances an individual's understanding of internal processes such as emotional responses and psychological patterns of our ego. The practice is an unwavering mirror.

In this respect, looking inward is not an "escape" but rather an engaged form of awareness. The classics sometimes refer to this attention as "lively stillness," that is, the body is still but the attention and focus is vigorously engaged.

Meditative practice can be broken down into four skills, all of which are necessary tools for developing and refining Qi:

1. cultivation of awareness

2. exploration and interrogation of the internal and external landscapes of the self

3. discovery of the streams of causation for the internal and external landscape

4. developing and sustaining calmness and tranquility.

Regulating the body and breath is an essential foundation for training the mind: the act of monitoring and adjusting the body and breath develops awareness of the chain of causation within the body as well as how the body and breath can be adjusted to develop a feeling of relaxation and ease. Song and structure of the body require attention, monitoring, and adjustments, all of which are acts of effort and concentration that strengthen awareness. The regulating of breath requires even more concentration and monitoring since both Buddhist and Taoist breathing techniques are not "natural" and must be ingrained into the body.

The body and breath are physical foundations upon which to strengthen the mind's will, focus, and discipline. That elevated awareness that begins with attention to the body and breath is refined until the mind can turn inward to interrogate its own processes. The body, breath, and mind exist in an interdependent loop, which feeds back upon itself (Figure 5.1). While on the surface the five regulations may appear to be stages—first body, then breath, then mind—since a person must fulfill the requirements for each before moving onto the next (i.e., body must be relaxed or breath cannot be directed). The entire process is more like a swirling circle than a ladder, where the regulation of one paves the way to understand and adjust the others. And within this circle, the mind is the central line around which the body and breath swirl in an infinite process of returning and building.

Breath

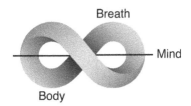

Mind

Body

FIGURE 5.1 THE DYNAMIC RELATIONSHIP
BETWEEN MIND, BODY, AND BREATH

The mind connects body and breath but is also the bridge to Qi and Shen. The mind adjusts body and breath and then harnesses that energy to refine it into Qi and Shen.

The Two Minds

The mind is sometimes referred to as the General or the Emperor because of its ability to direct, correct, and lead body, breath, and Qi. This "General" refers to "Yi" or intentional mind, which Western thinking would call the brain, the cognitive control center of the body, where the nervous system and organ functionality converge and are maintained. The term "brain" seems more appropriate in respect to neurocognitive processing since the input of sensory and ideational data is not only depersonalized but also treated as separate from other organ functionality. Yi, on the other hand, operates like a sensory organ such as the eyes, ears, nose, mouth, and skin: since data enter from the outside as sight, sound, smell, taste, and touch, the mind "senses" that information and reacts appropriately— sometimes unconsciously. Yet unlike the other senses, the mind has the unique capacity of shaping that response with a layering of emotional reaction and judgment (e.g., "That tastes good," "I like this," "I don't like that"). The Traditional Chinese Medicine view of the mind is less clinical and even recognizes a second mind, called "Xin" or emotional mind, which is the heart and the seat of emotional responses. Xin is the emotional center, whereas Yi is the intellectual center.

These two minds add a layer of further difficulty to training since Yi and Xin may not always be in synch with one another; and at worse, they are sometimes in opposition, which generates stress and anxiety. When we say that our heart is telling us one thing and our mind another, and we feel torn between the two, we are experiencing the fundamental split of the two minds, which suggests just how difficult regulating Yi and Xin can be. The place to begin, though, is with Song since that principle not only applies to body and breath but to mind as well.

Mind and Heart at Ease

Song resides at the heart of the saying "heart and mind at ease." After all, if the mind isn't calm, then the body and its Qi are not calm either. Since the mind is the governing agent that actively adjusts body and breath, a disturbed or troubled mind will be incapable of focusing on the body making the necessary adjustments. The emotional mind, Xin, is equally important since any emotional or psychological distress or excess will disrupt Yi, the body, and Qi. The slogan "The heart directs intention; intention directs movement" is extremely insightful in this respect. Emotions (Xin) alter perception (Yi), and those emotions will be transmitted to the physical body and breath, and will affect movement and breathing. The body and breath reveal the heart. To achieve a state of Song is not just physical relaxation and tranquil breathing but also penetrates past the surface to reach heart and mind. Emotional distress not only creates mental, physical, and respiratory tension, it also has health repercussions since each of the various organs are the sites for emotions according to the Five Elements Theory of Traditional Chinese Medicine. As detailed in

Table 5.1, each organ pertains to a specific emotion as well as a physical opening of the body and its sensory organ.

TABLE 5.1 THE FIVE ELEMENTS, THEIR ORGANS, AND EMOTIONS

ELEMENT	ORGAN	EMOTION	OPENING
Wood	Liver	Anger	Eyes
Fire	Heart	Joy	Ears
Earth	Spleen	Distress/worry	Mouth
Metal	Lung	Sadness/grief	Nose
Water	Kidney	Fear	Urethra/anus

Any emotional distress affects a particular organ and creates a Qi imbalance in that organ's meridians and channels.[16] Excessive emotions—even ones that are positive—impact the health of the body and drain energy. For example, long stints of laughter (joy/heart) are just as taxing to Qi as extended periods of weeping or anger. Laughing at a funny film or during conversations with a good friend often results in feeling tired. While emotions are not wrong, periods dominated by such emotions create imbalance in the body, which can be the seeds of disease and illness. The goal of "mind and heart at ease" is not to stifle emotions but to regulate excesses that are the sources of imbalance and potential health issues. Unchecked emotional extremes are to be avoided since they can spark disease. The result is to achieve a state of lasting calmness.

The relationship between emotions and organ health, as per Traditional Chinese Medicine, can be demonstrated through the impact of grief upon the health of the lungs. For example, when a spouse dies, it is not uncommon for the grieving widow or widower to become ill and sometimes die soon thereafter. Often one of the contributing factors in the death of the widowed spouse is pneumonia. The death of a loved one is extremely stressful, and that alone creates illness and physical distress, but the mourning process also includes immense grief, sadness, and crying. These emotions and physical responses correspond to the element of Metal and to the Lung. The emotional distress directly impacts the lungs, weakening them and making them more vulnerable to infection, such as the bacterial infection that can lead to pneumonia. If the widowed spouse is a less active elderly individual with a respiratory system that is already compromised by chronic obstructive pulmonary disease, blood pressure issues, or asthma, the lungs may not be capable of handling the added strain of grief and sadness. Such emotional stress is a contributing factor in the decline of an individual's health.

An emotional state is not the sole cause of a health condition or disease, but it is one of many possible contributing influences. Traditional Chinese Medicine considers three factors for disease: environment, lifestyle, and outlook. An emotional state falls within the category of outlook and directly impacts the Qi of the body and its organs by creating an imbalance. When Xin is tranquil and at ease, such imbalances are minimized, allowing for Yi to correct and adjust as necessary. The recipe for remaining healthy is to be measured and calm, as described in *Taoist Meditation*:

The energy in the body should not be scattered, the
spirit in the mind should not be dimmed.
How do you avoid scattering energy?
By not acting compulsively.
How do you avoid dimming the spirit?
By not keeping things on your mind.

(CLEARY 2000, P.III)

When both the mind and the heart are at ease, energy is not dispersed, and nothing is weighing upon Yi or Xin, the role of the Emperor/General can be performed with greater acumen thereby maintaining a sense of calmness and balance. Training the mind is absolutely central to the Qi of the body, which impacts all other aspects of health and well-being. As *Practical Taoism*, another Taoist classic, emphasizes, "Since energy comes from [the mind] opening, when the mind is harmonious the energy is harmonious, and when the energy is harmonious the body is harmonious. When the body is harmonious, the harmony of heaven and earth responds" (Cleary 1996, p.37). The centerpiece of health and well-being is a calm mind, and from that position of calmness, the mind can pursue the task of refining energy and cultivating Shen.

The Art of Tranquility

To achieve having the mind and heart at ease requires engaging in a process that is like a snake biting its own tail: to train the mind is to train the body; to train the body is to train the breath; to train the breath is to train the mind; and ad infinitum. Yet it is precisely the self-reflexive and inward turning of attention that leads to tranquility. The fundamental technique of adjusting the mind is known as "Yi Shou," or "keep the mind on." In Ch'an Buddhism, this technique is known as Single-Pointed Meditation, or "Staying and Returning," where the focus is directed to a specific spot, area, or process of the body, and when the practitioner notices that the attention has drifted from that point, focus is redirected back. The attention "stays," and when it has been distracted, it "returns" without judgment or commentary.[17] Sustained meditative practice strengthens the ability to concentrate and develop a more detailed awareness of the body and breath. This focused attention helps to illuminate the internal processes, causations, and triggers of the self, which might otherwise remain unconscious. How the body, breath, mind, and emotional state are connected in a chain of causation is brought into greater relief too: for example, a practitioner may discover where he or she holds stress in the body; or how the heart rate changes when confronted by a particular emotional trigger. Specific causes of tension, stress, and emotional responses are made clearer, and that understanding enables the individual to respond with even greater effectiveness to correct and harmonize.

The process of Yi Shou cultivates awareness, reveals connections, and makes the chain of causation of the self and its internal and external triggers more transparent and recognizable. In this respect, meditation is not a form of escapism where the indvidual retreats from the world; it is quite the opposite. This training brings into greater relief the internal and external landscapes so that the mind becomes more capable of making the necessary adjustments. In other words, a person will be able to see exactly where attention is being paid, and in doing so, will gain a more complete perspective of one's self. If thought returns to a specific issue or problem, for example, Yi Shou illuminates the state of the individual and where ideational energy is being directed. Without a clear perspective, the subtleties of where focus is being directed may remain buried. Energetically this is like having an unknown leaking water faucet: resources are being drained—slowly—and without the individual being aware of any depletion. Realizing how mental energy is being used allows for correction and redirection toward more healthy behaviors and patterns. To train the mind is to cultivate good, positive habits to replace bad, negative ones. The teachings of the Taoist "Pure Clarity of the Spiritual Jewel of the Exalted" in *Vitality, Energy, Spirit* offers a succinct and simple explanation:

> Practitioners should spy out the mind's habits, biases, prejudices, fixations, obsessions, and indulgences, so that eventually they can catch them and treat them accordingly. It will not do to be too easygoing; even slight faults should be eradicated, and even virtues should be developed. In this way entanglements may be cut off, and one may become constantly aware of true eternity. (Cleary 1991a, p.143)

These habits and flaws create an internal "dis-ease" that impacts the state of the practitioner. Furthermore, those flaws obscure the view of "true eternity." In other words, without regulating the habits and attachments of the mind, it is not possible to focus on spirituality; or to reframe this in terms of spirit and energy, the famous Taoist collection titled *Wen tzu* explains: "When the vitality, spirit, will, and energy are calm, they fill you day by day and make you strong. When they are hyperactive, they are depleted day by day, making you old" (Cleary 2003a, p.188). The state of the mind, whether agitated or calm, plays a pivotal role in the health of the individual as well as his or her Qi.

Training the mind requires a sustained self-reflective and self-reflexive awareness that is both an ability to observe and a willingness to investigate the whole self with all of its faults, flaws, shortcomings, and mistakes alongside all of the successes, triumphs, joys, and strengths. The texture of personhood is a complex fabric made up of positive and negative emotions, experiences, thoughts, and history, and the emotional layers of joy, guilt, anger, shame, regret, attachment, sadness, pride, and fear that overlay a self. To examine the complexities of personhood necessitates a strong, heroic attitude willing to examine the self with an unwavering and unflinching attention. The willingness to look at the self honestly and objectively leads to the ability to move from the base and into higher levels of human potential. As *The Book of Balance and Harmony* explains, the core practice depends on the ongoing refinement of the body, mind, and spirit.

The essential point in refining vitality is in the body…
The essential point in refining energy is in the mind.
The essential point in refining spirit is in the will.
(Cleary 2003b, p.412)

Mind bridges the vitality of the body and the spirit, but that refined Qi sustains the Will to Shen. Meditative practices strengthen the Will and seek to eliminate the negative things that impact the health of the body and that which derails the cultivation of Shen by perceiving the patterns and filters that obscure "true eternity." Yi Shou or Staying and Returning looks deeply in order to see through the veils and filters in order to discover the core self.

To arrive at a place of personal calmness, to whatever degree and for however long, is the core of training the mind. To remain calm in the face of any and all adversity is the mark of the sage and the ultimate goal of regulating mind. As the words carved above the entranceway to a small Taoist temple state so succinctly, "The recluse's heart is a placid lake unruffled by winds of circumstance." To train the mind is to cultivate a calmness that is unwavering in the face of adversity, and to harness energy that can be directed toward refining body, breath, and mind, and then transforming Qi into the source of Shen. "When body, mind and intent merge into one," according to the Taoist sourcebook *Vitality, Energy, Spirit*, "the vitality, energy, and spirit meet, without excitement or disharmony; this is the seed of the golden elixir" (Cleary 1991a, pp.142–143). The "golden elixir" is a harmonious union of being that is the source of the cultivation of Shen—higher spiritual consciousness and purpose. *The Secret of the Golden Flower*, another Taoist source, explains: "The turning around of the light is the 'firing process'" (Cleary 1991b, p.17). Yi Shou ignites the fire of Qi and provides the necessary energy to sustain the body, mind, and Shen.

Yi Feels, Discerns, Leads Qi

Previous discussions have shown the extent to which the mind works to ensure that the body is relaxed and properly structured so that the "furnace" is efficient, and that the breath is deep, long, slow, soft, equal, and tranquil, and that the Abdominal or Reverse Abdominal Breathing technique is utilized to maximize the "bellows" for Qi. The mind guides and adjusts these processes, but as we have seen, the mind not only can direct body and breath but also can lead Qi. A calm mind is a necessary condition to be able to properly execute the leading of Qi. As stated earlier, heart directs intention, and intention directs movement. That movement is both muscular as well as energetic. Any agitation, distraction, or emotional excess impacts Yi and Qi. A mind and heart at ease not only allows the attention to be undistracted and focused, it also allows for greater depth of feeling. The mind operates according to three distinct layers in relationship to monitoring and directing the body as well as Qi:

- feeling

- discerning

- leading.

To reach the ability to lead builds upon the skills of feeling and discerning, which need to be developed slowly and fully before attempting to leap forward into leading. The process of feeling tightness and looseness in the muscles and tendons, the flow and obstruction of Qi, harmony and imbalance, and empty and fullness in the body leads to the more precise identification of Yin and Yang in the body and its movements. Sensing the body more deeply and with greater precision enables the mind to discern and understand an issue, not just "feel" it. The mind's ability to lead emerges from the subtle depths of feeling and discernment: when the mind realizes blockages and imbalances, it can adjust the body and breath accordingly and appropriately in order to remove obstructions and harmonize flow. Discernment means being able to identify the source or root cause of the issue too, not just its physical manifestation. From that place of seeing, recognizing, and understanding, the mind can then direct Qi.

The sequencing of mind can be rendered in the following three stages of development:

1. mind alongside movement

2. mind inside movement

3. mind leading movement.

In the first step, the mind is an outside observer of the body, breath, and Qi—noticing and reacting after the fact to the feeling and movement of muscles, weight shifts, breath, and circulation. The mind, in this instance, adjusts retroactively. In the second step, the mind is actively engaged and its awareness is simultaneous with the movement. At this level, the mind discerns Yin and Yang of the body, breath, and Qi—instantaneously experiencing, identifiying, and correcting as each deviation occurs. In the final stage, the mind directs and is ahead of the movement, drawing Qi into different parts of body. Here the mind is the active catalyst that moves both the body and Qi. Each of these three steps happens at different times as well: mind alongside movement occurs *after* movement; mind inside movement happens *simultaneously*; and mind leading movement happens *before* a movement.

Feeling the body and breath, and then discerning these methods more acutely, is the focus of the previous two chapters (Chapters 3 and 4), and some of the exercises previously discussed show how leading is implicit within learning to use the tools of feeling and discerning. For example, the first posture of Da Mo's Wei Dan, where Qi is led to the palms, demonstrates the role of the mind as the agent for circulation. The visualization of engaging the muscles focuses Qi to flow to specific parts of the body. But in all of these examples, and even that of Wei Dan, the directing of Qi is an indirect by-product since the explicit mental focus is on the muscular movement and that movement sparks Qi by proxy.

Learning how to lead Qi is absolutely crucial to Qigong as well as Internal Martial Arts. A centerpiece of that training is often the classic Small Circulation (or Microcosmic) Breathing, wherein the mind is explicitly engaged in the process of feeling, discerning, and leading Qi. This technique is a mainstay in the development for regulating the mind and Qi.

The best way to practice Small Circulation Breathing is from a standing position with the feet shoulder width, and the body relaxed and aligned along the center standing pole. The tongue rests on the roof of the mouth, behind the front teeth, and touching the heart palate, which is slightly sensitive to the touch. The breath flows naturally in and out through the nose and adheres to the principles of deep, long, slow, soft, even, and tranquil. Abdominal/Buddhist Breathing is used to propel the breath and Qi, wherein the abdomen and Huiyin expand with inhalation, and relax and return to the neutral position with exhalation. Once the body achieves a state of Song, the mind and heart should release any residual tension. Take a few deep slow breaths to integrate body, breath, and mind, and feel the breath as deeply as possible.

The initial goal is to feel the Qi moving through the circuit—the Microcosmic Orbit—of the Governing Channel from the Dantian to the Huiyin, and then to the Mingmen and up the back to the Baihui, finishing beneath the nose and above the upper lip. Qi then flows through the Conception Channel from beneath the lower lip and down the front of the body to the Dantian. The tongue touching the heart palate bridges the gap between the two channels. The complete circuit makes a loop through the torso and head. The breath synchronizes with the flow of Qi by inhaling from the Dantian and up the Governing Channel and exhaling down the Conception Channel. (This breathing technique is discussed in Chapter 4.) The breath is used to facilitate the feeling of the two channels and to amplify the Qi moving through the Microcosmic Orbit. Qi is always coursing through this pathway, regardless of the mind's awareness or lack thereof, but the act of attention and awareness intensifies that flow.

This circuit of the linked Governing and Conception channels might be visualized as a string that is tied in a loop and then attached to two separate pegs—one at the crown of the head (Baihui) and the other between the legs (Huiyin). The loop of string circles continuously between these two pegs, but the act of mental attention creates an intensification of the movement through the channel. The mind, in this respect, is like a knot in the string where more mass is pushed through the circuit. The explicit goal is to feel the circuit and lead the Qi with intention. The mind feels the movement, discerns the flow through the channels, and directs that channel to flow with greater intensity through this specific causeway. Mastering this method translates into being able to direct Qi into specific parts of the body, which is used for releasing energy (Fajin) in Martial Arts training as well as directing Qi for the healing of self or others. The Small Circulation Breathing method enables the practitioner to understand the dynamic relationship of body, breath, mind, and Qi more intimately, and from the sensation of mind along with Qi and breath to mind inside Qi; and then, leading Qi through the Microcosmic Orbit, the mind can direct Qi for its transformation into Shen.

This technique can be found in numerous Taoist sources explicitly concerned with spiritual development. *Vitality, Energy, Spirit*, for example, refers to this as the "Three Passes," where the energy draws up the Governing Channel and its three vertebrae gates (or "Passes") of Mingmen (lower back), Shen Zhu (middle back), and the Jade Pillow (neck):

> *The body unmoving, refining vitality into energy,*
> *   rising through the coccyx, is called the first pass.*
> *The mind unmoving, refining energy into spirit,*
> *   stopping at midspine, is called the middle pass.*
> *The intent unmoving, refining spirit into spaciousness,*
> *   rising to the back of the skull, is called the upper pass.*
>
> (CLEARY 1991A, PP.142–143)

Drawing Qi through the Microcosmic Orbit enhances the role of the mind in relation to body, breath, and Qi: the mind learns how to sense Qi, discern the quantity and quality of Qi as well as potential obstructions for the harmonious flow of Qi (muscular tightness, constriction, improper breath, and so forth), and guides energy through the channels to specific parts of the body. The same sequencing is found in more advanced techniques such as Embryonic Breathing, where the Qi is directed through the thrusting channel and along the Water path to connect the lower and upper Dantians and in order to open the Mud Pill Palace—the seat of higher spiritual consciousness located in the cerebral cortex. The training process involves locating and feeling the lower, middle, and upper Dantians, as well as the Thrusting Channel that connects them; discerning the pathway and any blockages along that channel; leading the breath and Qi to fill the lower and then upper Dantian; and then drawing Qi from the lower Dantian into the Mud Pill Palace in order to open the seat of higher consciousness and refine energy into Shen.[18]

All of these methods, from simple and fundamental meditative practices to the most advanced and complex forms of meditative Qigong, train the mind to feel, discern, and lead. And all emphasize principles that apply equally to body, breath, and mind:

- Body, breath, and mind must be relaxed and at ease (Song).

- The flow of movement whether of the physical body, the breath, or thought should be smooth, even, and harmonious.

- The entire process should be self-reflexive and governed by a sense of tranquil, objective awareness ("lively stillness") that monitors, corrects, and maintains the self.

These three applied principles shape the quantity, quality, and flow of Qi as well:

- When the body, breath, and mind are calm, the Qi is tranquil and not dispersed.

- When movement is even and not agitated, the flow of Qi is smooth.

- When the body, breath, and mind are united through concentrated awareness, Qi is amplified, refined, and can be directed for specific purposes.

Vitality, Energy, Spirit refers to this process of integrating body, breath, mind, and Qi as the "Five Energies Returning to the Origin":

> *The five energies are the true energies of*
> *the five fundamental forces.*
> *When they are correctly aligned they congeal into one.*
> *When your body is not agitated, your vitality is*
> *stable, and its energy returns to the origin.*
> *When your mind is not agitated, your breath is*
> *stable, and its energy returns to the origin.*
> *When your nature is always tranquil, the higher soul*
> *is stored, and its energy returns to the origin.*
> *When emotions are forgotten, the lower soul is*
> *subdued, and its energy returns to the origin.*
> *When physically elements are in harmony, the will*
> *is stable, and its energy returns to the origin.*

When these five forces are in their proper
place and at peace, they revert to their
reality, which is the source of religion.

(CLEARY 1991A, P.142)

These five elements and their energies are the body, mind, character, emotion, and the overall health and well-being of the self. When the body, breath, and mind unite in a state of subdued tranquility, the Source of life and the way of Shen can be perceived more clearly. Different traditions have various names for this Source—Buddha mind, original nature, and Tao, for example—but the path to discover that Source must travel through the cultivation, refinement, and concentration of self and Qi. Energy is the bridge between the Source and the body, breath, and mind. Qi flows from the Source, and in order to trace it back, the mind must be cultivated and made more sensitive. The path to the Source is revealed only by refining the self. The regulation of body, breath, mind, Qi, and Shen is a progression of cultivation of the individual, wherein the body leads to breath, the breath leads to mind, the mind leads to Qi, and all of these meld together into the spirit, the Qi of Shen.

"Duo zhu yi yang shen" is a classic training slogan that translates as "Pay attention to nurturing." The way of nurturing is the path of cultivation of self with its energy, vitality, and spirit. The means by which such nurturing happens is through the active role of the mind to concentrate on the internal landscape of the self—the body and breath as well as its internal processes—as well as the external landscape—the world one must navigate with all of its people, things, and happenings. The mind negotiates the intersection of the internal and the external. Refining the mind is a refinement of perception since the state of mind—whether agitated or calm—colors how the self and the world are perceived. The mind holds the key. To reach enlightenment, the "original mind" is awakened. In Taoism, the sage reaches a state of what the *Tao Te Ching* calls "no fixed mind" wherein the mind is able to ebb and flow with the Tao, thereby always being part of its stream with no restrictions, no contention, and no disruptions. The ultimate goal is a mind that is unobstructed, calm, abiding, and free from attachments. To nurture such a mind refines the energy into Shen and uses that energy to return to the Source.

Cultivating a Garden

The classic terms for the relationship of body, breath, and mind is furnace, bellows, and cauldron. Such an analogy with the mind/cauldron steaming and boiling is a wonderful image of spiritual work where the practice is a continuous and sustained process of self-cultivation. The image of the boiling cauldron is extremely applicable for a monastic setting in that every aspect of monastic life fuels the dedication to spiritual pursuits. Meditation, chanting, study, recitation, work, ritual, and more provide nonstop tools for the act of "steaming the mind." At one of the monasteries where I stayed there were even signs in the bathrooms that read "As I eliminate this waste from my body, may I also eliminate attachments and desires." Every moment and every activity sparks the regulation of Shen. A monastery, in this respect, is a very rarified environment that is specially designed to manifest Shen—spiritual consciouness and awakening.

Outside of the walls of a monastery, in the secular world, the same opportunities to continuously stoke the spiritual fire of the mind may not be as frequent. Familial and social responsibilities, work obligations, and navitating a world where the goals, purposes, and values of others may contrast with our spiritual pursuits creates difficulties for personal cultivation. Such difficulties are minimized in a monastic setting. In the secular world it takes extra effort to carve out the time and space from social, familial, and work responsibilities for spiritual cultivation; consequently, practice may seem to be part-time and progress slow to actualize. It is still possible to pay attention to nurturing Shen, but given the gradual pace of progress and that it is difficult to dedicate every moment to spiritual life, training cannot happen with the same constant intensity as in a monastery. The approach needs to be more open in order to be responsive to the demands of a secular life. In this respect, the training is more akin to gardening than constantly boiling a cauldron.

The natural world doesn't require tending in order for plants, trees, and flowers to grow. This process happens without our interference. In the same way, the body, breath, and mind continue without the need to "pay attention to nurturing." Yet the sustained cultivation of the self sparks deeper growth. Like an untended field with wild plants, flowers, trees, or grain, Qi continues to sustain life without oversight, but with proper tending, a field can be transformed into a properous and highly sustainable farm, and a wild bunch of flowers can become a cultivated garden with overflowing beauty. That garden requires ongoing tending and cultivation, though, in order to be maintained.

The image of a manicured garden may not seem to accord with the Tao since a central lesson of abiding is to let things happen naturally without undue interference. After all, when we interfere, we create resistance, which generates problems (i.e., "dis-ease"). Lao Tzu states that "only by non-contention is there nothing extreme" (Cleary 1992, p.12). To contend is to interfere, which disrupts the natural flow and creates imbalance. An accomplished gardener or farmer does abide by the Tao since he or she understands that things will grow only if they are planted in harmony with the natural cycle of the year and in a climate that matches the nature of the plant. Western American culture, too, has its Tao of planting and harvesting. The idea of acting in accord with the natural world is the governing principle behind *The Farmer's Almanac*, a sourcebook for gardeners and farmers concerning when and how to plant, grow, and harvest throughout the year, and to be a successful garderner is to understand and respect this natural cycle.

The comparison with the natural world is to think of ourselves as soil, seeds, and a gardener. The body is the soil that is tended, so it is more fertile for the seeds of energy to grow. The breath provides the sustenance—the air and nutrients—that spark growth of the seeds. The mind is the gardener that oversees the entire process by watering, adding fertilizer, trimming, weeding, and supporting in order to maximize growth. The gardener adjusts and culls in response to the situation and nurtures for future growth. In the same way, we work with what is already there and do not interfere with the natural process since such intrusion is the source of tension, stress, and disease. Like a conscientious gardener, we prepare and maintain ourselves with proper nutrients and lifestyles, we plant the seeds that we nurture and grow, and we nourish those seeds with our breath. Throughout the process, the mind tends and adjusts accordingly so that growth and progress is maintained. Nurturing the self cannot be neglected or performed sporadically. The awareness and focus needs to be steady and regular since growth happens only with vigilant effort and Will.

Since the Dantian is also known as "Energy Seed Field," the parallel between nurturing a garden and Qi, Jing, and Shen is extremely apt. But what exactly are we growing? What are the seeds that we plant, nourish, and tend? Obviously it is Qi, but that Qi fuels a number of purposes:

- health of body and mind

- well-being

- calmness and tranquilty

- a connectedness to ourselves and our world.

The cultivation of Qi ultimately reinforces the relationship between ourselves and the world. It is the trace that brings us back to our origin where we are in accord with the natural flow of life. We return to our fundamental selves, and every opportunity that life presents, whether as an obstacle, a detour, or a celebration, is a way to deepen our understanding of that essential self. To cultivate Qi is to embark upon the never-ending path of energy, vitality, and spirit, a path that embraces Qi, Jing, and Shen as the foundations and the tools for living a life that reaps the fullness of the Tao.

CHAPTER 6

The Elements of Daily Practice

Grandmaster William C.C. Chen grinned broadly when he heard the question—as if he was waiting for just this moment. "How much should I practice?" floated from the back of the seminar room, and the eyes of seventy or so people shifted to Grandmaster Chen as he began to answer.

"You should practice at least twenty minutes every day." Then he paused as if reconsidering, and added, "But on those days when you are so busy…(again, a pause) on those days, practice at least two hours."

The people in the audience hesitated, and then a few people began to laugh as Grandmaster Chen's eyes lit up and a huge smile erupted on his face. The room then filled with laughter. His answer and its delivery were masterful, but the issues of how much and how often to practice frequently come up in any discussion of Internal Arts, and like Grandmaster Chen, I encourage people to adopt a daily routine so that their practice can become integrated into their lives. I frequently warn beginners that many of them start this practice in order to remedy stress, and the amount of their practice shouldn't be a source of more stress for them. Yet one of my favorite sayings is extremely relevant: "Good medicine tastes bitter." Effort is necessary to make positive changes, even if the act of making positive changes is discomforting and difficult.

During a service at a church in Pittsburgh, a Ch'an Buddhist abbot was asked to talk about Buddhism and meditation. He offered meditation instruction to the congregation, and led them through an abbreviated Ch'an service. At the end of the church service, he asked if anyone had any questions or comments. A number of people did, but one in particular has stuck with me for ten years or more. A man remarked, "The meditation was great, but I just don't have time to meditate every day." The abbot replied in typical Ch'an matter-of-factness, "So on days you are really busy, you don't go to the bathroom?" His reply was met with a steely silence.

Necessary Medicine

Practice needs to be approached with discipline and dedication—and as a *need* and not a hobby. Everyone's life is busy. Everyone has stress. Taking time for personal cultivation may seem indulgent, yet the exact opposite is true. When we retreat into ourselves and nourish ourselves, we are better equipped to deal with everything that life presents to us: deadlines, arguments, tension, and responsibilities become manageable; and the joyous, celebratory moments become even more so.

Master Yang Yang has a wonderful way of rendering the importance of practice in relationship to life. He emphasizes practice as the following equation: $10 - 1 > 10$.

Mathematically this does not compute, but the gist is that if there are ten hours of work to address, taking one hour out of that ten to practice translates into it seeming as if there are more than ten hours left in which to take care of what requires one's attention. The result, though, is qualitative and not quantitative, and the increase in focus and energy that comes with regular practice isn't measured in gained hours but in the ability to do better, more efficient work—and perhaps even a sense that the various tasks are an integral part of daily life instead of a disruption.

This is also the gist of Grandmaster Chen's wry response that on really busy days a person should practice even more than usual because the added focus and energy is needed even more; or, practice more, work better. The end point is achieving a sense of balance and practicing well.

But not all practice is equal. A classic maxim is "The most important thing in learning Martial Arts is to practice in the proper way." In order to maximize results and gain more, training needs to have focus and purpose. Energy, vitality, and spirit should drive practice forward—invigorating it and giving it direction. When we approach practice we should keep in mind that we are working toward goals that we set for ourselves, and while the specific nature of those goals are for each person to define, they ultimately should touch upon three areas:

- cultivation of physical health and well-being

- balancing of the emotional and psychological aspects of self

- affirmation of place and purpose in the world at large.

Ultimately, the practice navigates internal and external spaces—the fabric of the self and the world at large.

It is not the intention of this book to be dogmatic and tell people what to practice or why, but rather to point toward the great potential that this path can make manifest. The discovery of *why* a person trains is for him or her to find out.

The way of cultivating and discovering the self, though, requires constant energy and a daily routine that not only keeps the individual moving on the path but one that gradually and continuously cultivates Qi, Jing, and Shen to sustain the practitioner. How Qi, Jing, and Shen is applied to living is up to each person since energy, vitality, and spirit can be nurtured for the Martial Arts, healing, thinking, teaching, or as the fuel to become a "Real Human," or even a combination of any or all of these things. There is no set end result or even one path when it comes to waking up, tapping Buddha mind, discovering infinite happiness, or floating effortlessly in the stream of the Tao. But a person needs energy and vitality, and spiritual focus, to stay on the path and achieve the goal.

What follows is an overview of the fundamental elements of a daily practice with the explicit goal of creating a united body, breath, mind, and Qi. An individual does not need to do all of these exercises in order to cultivate energy, vitality, and spirit, and other methods may be just as effective, but presented here is what has been handed down through many generations of teachers and masters, which I have interpreted, modified, and presented. All of these methods have withstood the test of time—some for thousands of years—as being extremely effective and safe. As with any physical exercise, though, it is best to consult a doctor before engaging in any type of exercise regime to make sure that it is appropriate for the individual's physical condition and health. I have tried to be as detailed and precise as possible in the discussion of the exercises that follows, but a book by its very nature pales in comparison to working with a teacher. These exercises are the beginnings of an energetic practice, and that practice would be greatly enhanced by finding a qualified master to work with directly.

Daily Practices

Wuji Standing Meditation

Wuji Standing Meditation, also known as "Embracing the Tree," is an ancient form of Standing Taoist Meditation, and within Chen-style Taiji practice, it is regarded as a "closed" secret. Wuji Meditation was taught along with San Ti (Three Poles) Standing Meditation to what are known as "inside students"—those people whom teachers would invite into a studio or home to train. "Outside students" would be those who might train, but in a less intimate, public setting, such as a park, with limited instruction. Wuji was an important training technique reserved for select students. Since 2000, Wuji Standing has become available outside of these closed circles, but its importance is in no way diminished. The term "Wuji" means "no polarity" and refers to the complete harmony prior to Yin and Yang. The name helps to reveal the feeling behind the technique; that is, the practitioner achieves a state of harmonious balance where weight is equally dispersed, stance is solid, and mind, heart, and body are relaxed.

There are various styles of Wuji Standing Meditation including: (a) Holding Ball (or Three Circle); (b) Raising Ball, Pressing Ball, and Lifting Ball; and (c) Resting. The focus here is on the Holding Ball style of standing. The standing posture adheres to basic Standing Post Qigong (Figure 6.1):

1. Feet are shoulder width with the toes either parallel or turning slightly outward.

2. Knees are open with a slight natural bend.

3. Hips and waist are soft allowing the weight of the body to be released downward into the ground.

4. Shoulders are relaxed with slightly bent elbows and soft hands and fingers slightly curved.

5. The center of the chest (sternum) is hollowed slightly allowing the diaphragm to relax downward.

6. Chin is tucked in slightly, bringing the neck and head in alignment with the spine.

7. The top of the head is suspended upward.

8. Tongue is on the roof of the mouth, behind the top teeth, touching the heart palate.

9. Breathing is in and through the nose using Abdominal/Buddhist Breathing.

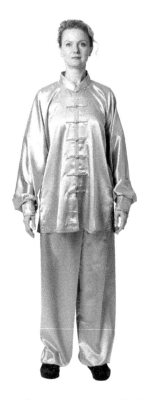

FIGURE 6.1 STANDING POST QIGONG

The stance is stuctured like a post in the ground: aligned, rooted, and erect. The stance should feel natural with the body in comfortable alignment. There are two sayings that help bring the body into proper stance. The first saying is "Imagine that you are one inch taller"; the other is "Listen behind you." Once the body is in proper position, the breathing can be deep, long, slow, soft, even, and tranquil, and the mind can be serene.

To perform Wuji Standing Meditation, first align oneself in the Standing Post Qigong, then with the feeling of the toes gripping the ground, lift the arms as if holding a ball in front of the chest (Figure 6.2). The hands are soft and relaxed with the fingers slightly separated from one another and curved inward. The palms of the hands face inward toward the chest and are approximately one foot from the chest. A space of approximately six inches separates the hands. The shoulders are relaxed, arm pits are open, and elbows are slightly bent and soft. There should not be any tension in the chest, back, shoulders, and arms. The tongue rests on the heart palate, and breathing is in and out through the nose following Abdominal or Buddhist Breathing. The focus of the mind is on the Dantian— watching, observing, and feeling. The gaze is directed at the space between the hands.

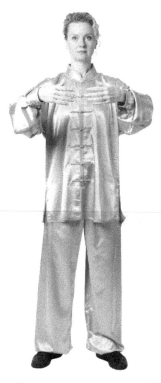

FIGURE 6.2 WUJI STANDING MEDITATION

When a person first begins the meditation, use a timer so that the attention does not need to shift back and forth watching a clock. Initially start with three minutes. If that meditation time passes without undue physical strain and mental distraction for one week, then add one minute to the session. Increase the amount of time spent in Wuji Meditation gradually and as a response to what feels natural. The amount of time in Wuji need not exceed twenty minutes, but it should be performed once a day.

The objective of Wuji Meditation is to unite body, breath, and mind naturally—not through force. Simply allow the body, breath, and mind to relax and merge together.

Kaimen Qigong Meditation

"Kaimen" in Chinese means to open a door, and as a Qigong form it refers to Opening the Gates of the Body. Kaimen Meditation is an ancient Taoist form of Qigong that integrates body, breath, and mind in order to lead Qi through the energetic channels of the body (Figure 6.3). The simple exercise is performed slowly with the cadence of the breath matched to the movement of the hands. Doing Kaimen Qigong after performing Wuji Standing Meditation is ideal, and the exercise should be performed regularly on a daily basis.

To begin, align the body in the Standing Pole Qigong position with the hands relaxed at the sides of the body (see Figure 6.1). Allow the mind and heart to relax and extend the depth of feeling inward. Breathe soft, deep, natural breaths into the abdomen using Abdominal or Buddhist Breathing. Once the body is relaxed and the breath is natural, turn the palms of both hands forward and lift the palms upward slightly to the front of the body. Inhale as the palms continue up over the head and then arc the arms with the palms facing downward as if holding a ball that is balanced on top of the head. The hands begin to descend toward Baihui (Heaven's Cap) at the crown of the head and then continue down the front of the face to the throat, chest, and lower Dantian, and then return to the starting position at the sides of the body. Exhale as the hands descend from the top of the head to the starting position. The movement of the hands and the exhalation facilitate the flow of Qi through the front of the body, which is amplified by mental concentration. The mind leads the Qi alongside the hands, in the following pathway:

1. From the Baihui, split the Qi to flow down the sides of the face, then unite the two paths into one at the top of the throat.

2. Direct the Qi to the top of the chest, where it splits again and travels in two paths to the outside of the nipples and then back toward the center of the chest, where it makes a complete circle that merges again at the diaphragm.

3. The pathway then descends to the Dantian and to Huiyin, where the Qi splits one last time to travel down the inside (Yin channels) of the legs to Yongquan ("Bubbling Wells" in the feet) and into the ground.

The visualization of Qi flowing downward to Huiyin takes place with the hands descending to the sides. The hands rest at the sides as the mind directs the flow down the Yin channel of the legs.

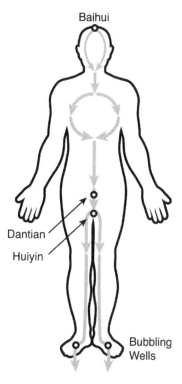

Baihui

Dantian

Huiyin

Bubbling
Wells

FIGURE 6.3 KAIMEN QIGONG

The entire sequence uses one breath cycle, with the Qi leading from the Baihui to Yongquan and into the ground occurring with the exhalation. If it is difficult to feel the flow of Qi down the body, multiple breath cycles can be used to enhance the exercise. Where the feeling of the channel is lost or uncertain, complete the exhalation, then inhale softly, initiating the sequence again from that stopping point. The inhalation increases the Qi and enhances the ability to sense the flow in the channel. The entire exercise should be repeated nine times.

Kaimen creates a bridge between body, breath, mind, and Qi, and the benefits not only include generating more Qi as well as creating a more harmonious flow of Qi within the body, but also creating a sense of meditative tranquility and well-being.

Still Mountain (Jing Shan) Qigong

Qigong, which translates as "energy work," is one of the most effective strategies of integrating body, breath, and mind, and working with Qi and Shen. Still Mountain (Jing Shan) Qigong is a set that has grown out of my own background in Traditional Chinese Medicine, Buddhist and Taoist philosophy and practice, as well as my decades of training in Internal Arts, and it is the namesake set that I teach at my studio (Still Mountain T'ai Chi and Chi Kung). The saying in Taiji is that it should be "Still as a mountain and flow like a river." "Jing" means both "still" and "tranquil," and "Shan" is "mountain." The essence of the set is for the body and mind to be a still, tranquil mountain—but one vibrant with Qi coursing like a river through the entire body. Jing in this respect refers to the principles of the body, breath, and mind being relaxed, rooted, and focused, and the movements are soft, flowing, and harmonious.

A few basics are as follows:

- The stance is Standing Pole Qigong, with slight deviations for the placement of feet in Touching

Heaven and Earth (posture 3), which uses an empty stance, and Turn the Windlass to Circulate Qi (posture 4), which uses a classic bow stance.

- The breathing uses Abdominal or Buddhist Breathing.

- Each of the moves should be repeated eight times.

- Each posture strives to integrate physical movement, breath sequencing, and mental application into a unified whole.

Posture 1: Preparation

Align the body in the Standing Pole Qigong posture and soften knees, hips, waist, shoulders, elbows, and hands. The center of the chest in the middle Dantian should be relaxed and hollowed. Tuck the chin in slightly and lengthen the neck by drawing the head upward from inside the body. Allow the weight to sink to the feet and root into the ground. Once the root is established, gently rock forward and backward without lifting the heels or toes. The feet should remain flat on the ground during rocking. Use a deep, long, slow, and soft breath in coordination with the rocking. Breathing should be Abdominal or Buddhist Breathing.

MENTAL APPLICATION

Mental focus should be directed inward; that is, feeling the stance and determining if there is any residual physical tension or discomfort in the body, and, if there is, allowing that tension to dissolve, be released, and flow into the ground through the body and feet. The attention is fixed upon feeling the body and discerning its Yin and Yang aspects.

Posture 2: Hands Lift to Awaken Qi

Begin from the Standing Pole Qigong position with hands resting at the sides of the body; the hands then raise to waist level with the palms facing upward as if the hands are under an object and holding it in front of the body (Figure 6.4A). Inhale as the hands lift up the front of the body to the sternum or middle Dantian, and exhale as the hands rotate, palms down, and descend back to the starting position at the waist (Figure 6.4B). Inhale again and rotate and raise the palms along the front of the body and over the head (Figure 6.4C). The gaze follows the hands as they move upward. The hands then separate to the left and right, descending in arcs away and down back to the sides of the legs (Figure 6.4D). As the hands descend to the sides, exhale. Bring the hands palms up back to the waist level, and repeat for a total of eight times.

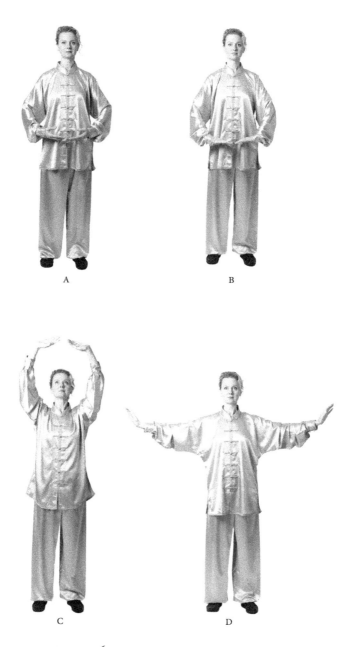

FIGURE 6.4A–D HANDS LIFT TO AWAKEN QI

MENTAL APPLICATION

The mind directs Qi up the Thrusting Channel from the Dantian, to the middle Dantian, and then up through the Baihui and over the head. Lead Qi down the front of the body along the Conception Channel back to the Dantian as the arms descend down the sides to the starting position. Qi moves in a circle up the Thrusting Channel and down the Conception Channel to the Dantian.

Posture 3: Touching Heaven and Earth

The posture begins in the Standing Pole stance with the hands at sternum level with the palms facing toward one another (Figure 6.5A). The hands are separated from one another by the few inches and are approximately six inches in front of the body. The left hand lifts upward and over the head with the palm facing toward the sky and the fingers pointing in toward the body (Figure 6.5B). The hand position is slightly in front of the body. As the left hand lifts, the right hand descends to waist level with the palm facing down to the ground and the fingers pointed forward and away from the body. Both left and right arms are extended but do not lock the shoulders, elbows, or wrists. As the arms begin to move (left hand lifting to touch heaven, right hand descending to touch earth), shift the weight onto the left leg and step the right foot forward about eight inches in front with the right toe lightly touching the ground in an empty stance. The weight of the body is on the left leg, but do not lock the hip, knee, or ankle of the left leg, and be careful not to lean to either side.

As the hands lift and the foot steps forward to touch the toe, inhale. Hold the position, then exhale naturally, and inhale once more. With the second exhale, drop the left elbow and draw down the left hand. The right hand draws up to the chest as the left hand descends, with both hands returning to face palm to palm at the middle Dantian. As the hands move, step back with the right leg and shift the weight onto it. The posture now switches to the other side with the right hand extending upward, left hand down, and the left leg stepping forward. Inhaling as the hands and leg move into the posture, exhale gently holding the position, then inhale again, and then exhale to return to the starting position with hands at chest level.

Repeat the entire sequence of both sides eight times.

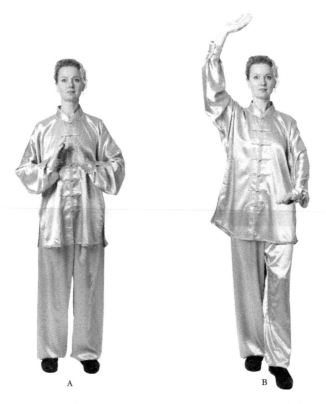

A   B

FIGURE 6.5A AND B TOUCHING HEAVEN AND EARTH

MENTAL APPLICATION

Qi is directed from the Dantian through the channels of the arms and legs. As the hands and leg move, lead Qi from the Dantian to bridge the arms and legs. While holding the posture with the breath cycle, connect the limbs and direct energy to flow to the gates of the palms ("Labor Valley") and balls of the feet ("Bubbling Wells"). As the leg steps back in and the hands return to the chest, lead Qi back to the Dantian.

Posture 4: Turn the Windlass to Circulate Qi

The posture begins from the Standing Post position, then turn the right foot slightly (30 degrees from center), shift the weight onto the right foot, bring the left toe next to the instep of the right foot into an "empty T" stance, then step the left foot about twelve inches forward with the toes pointed straight forward in a classic bow stance (Figure 6.6A). The weight of the body is on the back right leg, and the palms are parallel to the ground about waist high. The hands draw back toward the body and then up the front of the body to chest height, and then make loose fists. Push the fists forward while shifting the weight onto the front leg (Figure 6.6B). Open the hands as they circle down and back toward the body again; the weight again shifts onto the back leg. The motion is like rowing a boat or turning a windlass. As the hands draw up the body, inhale; as the fists push forward, exhale. Repeat the movement eight times, and then switch sides so that the right leg is forward and the left leg is back in the bow stance. Repeat this sequence eight times on the right side.

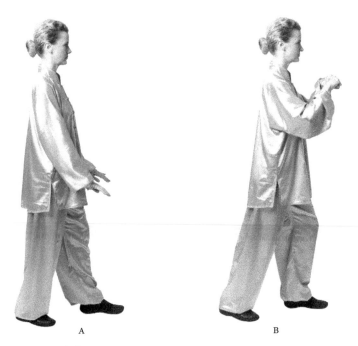

A   B

FIGURE 6.6A AND B TURN THE WINDLASS TO CIRCULATE QI

MENTAL APPLICATION

As the hands draw up the front of the body, visualize Qi drawing up from the feet and into the back. The Qi then is directed into the arms and fists with the exhalation and forward motion. As the hands descend down to circle again, the Qi circles the front of the body and to the ground. The Qi circulation mirrors the circular physical movement. As the arms make a small circle, the Qi is making a larger circle up the legs, through the Governing Channel, down the Conception Channel, and down the legs.

Posture 5: Picking Stars and Circling the Earth

The arms begin relaxed at the sides of the body, and the stance is Standing Post (Figure 6.1). Bring the left hand palm up to the Dantian (Figure 6.7A). The right hand stays relaxed and still. Lift the left palm a few inches in front of the body. When the palm reaches the eyes, rotate the hand so that palm is now facing the sky. Continue moving the palm upward as the eyes follow the path of the hand (Figure 6.7B). Turn the body to the right and arc the left hand down toward the floor (Figure 6.7C). The waist bends as the hand reaches toward the floor palm down, and the knees stay open but not bent (Figure 6.7D). Once the hand reaches the body's maximum stretch without overexerting, circle the hand along the floor palm down to the left side, as if drawing a semicircle on the ground (Figure 6.7E). Once the hand reaches the left side, turn the palm up, straighten the waist, and lift the hand back over the head (Figure 6.7F). To finish, lead the palm down the front of the body.

Inhale as the hand lifts over the head, and exhale as the body turns and the hand descends to the floor and draws the arc. Inhale as the body straightens and the hand rises over the head, and exhale as the palm leads down the front of the body.

The arms alternate to make eight total repetitions, so after the left hand circles and the right hand leads up over the head, turn the body opposite to the left side, lead down, arc around the floor to the right, lift up, and then the right hand descends. The entire sequence makes a large circle around the body starting and ending over the head.

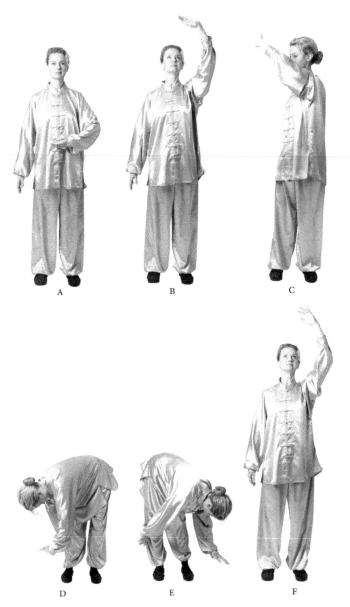

FIGURE 6.7A–F PICKING STARS AND CIRCLING THE EARTH

MENTAL APPLICATION

As the hand lifts along the front of the body, lead Qi from Dantian to Baihui through the Thrusting Channel. Concentrate on directing Qi to the palms, feet, and crown of the head. In the final part of the movement when the palm descends back down the front of the body, the mind draws Qi into the Baihui and leads it into the Dantian.

Posture 6: Gather Qi

Begin with the palms facing in toward the body, waist level, with the hands about one and a half feet away from the body, as if holding a beachball against the front of the abdomen. The feet are shoulder width and the body is in Standing Pole stance with the waist slightly bent and the body leaning forward as if reaching for something across a table (Figures 6.8A and 6.8B). Draw the palms toward the Dantian (Figure 6.8C). When the hands are a few inches in front of the abdomen, pull the elbows out and away from the body and rotate the arms around as if the hands are turning around to gather and embrace and in doing so returning to the starting position of holding the ball (Figure 6.8D). Inhale as the hands draw in to the Dantian, and exhale as the hands circle back to front (Figure 6.8A).

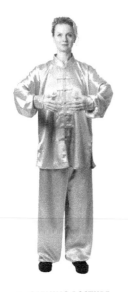

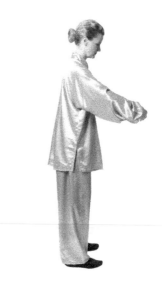

A. OPENING POSTURE

B. OPENING POSTURE SIDE VIEW

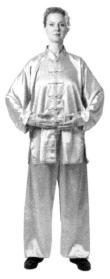

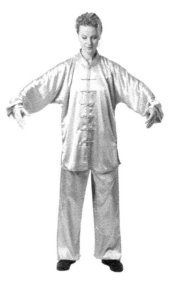

C. DRAWING QI INTO DANTIAN
WITH THE HANDS

D. TURN ELBOWS AND ROTATE HANDS TO
RETURN TO THE OPENING POSTURE

FIGURE 6.8A–D GATHER QI

MENTAL APPLICATION

Draw Qi into the Dantian to store as the hands come toward the abdomen. As the hands circle back out, release surplus energy through the arms, wrists, and fingertips, then visualize gathering Qi from outside of the body to pull into the body to store.

Posture 7: Closing Visualization

In the Standing Post stance, close the eyes, and starting from the top of the head, slowly bring the attention down through the body, letting any discovered tension, tightness, or physical, emotional, or psychological discomfort dissolve and flow down to the feet and into the ground. Allow the entire body inside and out to soften and relax as if standing in a shower and the warm water is cascading over the body and carrying with it any problems, sickness, or disease. Visualize that the crown of the head, the Baihui, is open, and Qi is flowing into the head, slowly pouring into every part of the body and flowing to the Dantian, which sits like a large bowl collecting the Qi. Once the bowl fills, imagine the Qi overflowing and streaming down the inside of the legs to the feet and into the ground. At this point Qi is flowing continuously into the top of the head, through the body, and into the ground.

To finish, slowly open the eyes, rock the weight from side to side, front to back, and then gently lift the feet.

Seated Meditation

The art of meditation is not hard to learn, but it requires effort to master. The Ch'an practice called Single-Pointed Meditation (Yi Shou) is a way of training the mind, cultivating spiritual development, and healing oneself both physically and psychologically.

First, find a place that is quiet and with few distractions. The environment should not be filled with things that will attract the senses or spark the mind to ruminate and reflect, since the goal is to develop sustained and focused awareness. Use a chair, kneeling bench, or a cushion, and take care that the body is properly aligned so that physical discomfort is minimized and the circulatory paths of the body remain open to maintain the flow of the body's Qi.

The proper structure of the body is built upon a tripod of both feet flat on the ground and the tailbone in the center of the seat (if sitting on a chair) or both knees against a mat or the floor and the tailbone in the center of the bench or cushion. The weight should be more or less equal between the knees and tailbone so that the feet do not fall asleep.

The spine should be straight but relaxed. In order to bring the spine into alignment, press the navel forward and the tailbone tucks under the body. Do not straighten the back by raising the shoulders since this creates tension in the lower back and between the shoulder blades. The shoulders should remain relaxed, and the chin should be tucked slightly inward but parallel with the shoulders. The tongue rests behind the top front teeth on the roof of the mouth at the heart palate, and the breath, which is silent and relaxed, flows in and out through the nose. The eyes should remain open but unfocused. With the chin parallel with the shoulders, the gaze should drop to no more than three or four feet to the ground in front.

Finally, the hands should rest about two-thirds of the way down the legs in a meditative mudra with the thumb of both hands covering the nails of the index finger known as "Closing the Tiger's Mouth." The hand, in this position, forms an "OK" sign and the backs of the hands rest on the thighs.

Once the body is properly aligned, the mind focuses on the Dantian. This form of meditation is called Single-Pointed (Yi Shou) Meditation and consists of the mind remaining focused on the Dantian through the process of staying and returning. The goal is to maintain focus and, as various body sensations or thoughts arise, to bring the attention back to the Dantian, thereby training the mind to remain focused through the process of "staying and returning."

Sit for fifteen to thirty minutes depending on the amount of time one's schedule allows. Also, try to establish a daily routine in order to maximize the physical and psychological benefits of meditation.

Meditative Reflections

Daily practice should not only train body, breath, and Qi, but needs to include mind and heart (Yi and Xin). Directed meditation is one such way to address the issues that impact emotionality and psychology of the self in order to gain clarity about oneself and reach a state of self-awareness and tranquil acceptance. An effective form of meditative inquiry is to use a saying as a tool to interrogate the self. One such saying is "Everyone is in search of his or her best interests and happiness."

This reflection should take place in a quiet environment so as not to be disturbed. The best posture is the seated position described in the instructions for Single-Pointed Meditation (see above), although the hands can simply rest palms down on the thighs instead of in the Tiger's Mouth mudra. The object of the meditation is to apply the saying that "everyone works for his or her best interest and happiness" to a life event. For example, the saying can be applied to an interaction with another person where that individual said or did something like cutting ahead in traffic or in a queue at the store. Reflecting on the saying helps to illuminate the social dynamic of the pursuit of self-satisfaction—not as a form of judgment of others but as a way of contextualizing intentionality and motives. That understanding of others needs to be applied to oneself as well. The directed meditation needs to investigate an instance in one's own life to see how that experience was self-motivated by personal interest as well.

The goal of this meditation is not to judge others or oneself for certain behaviors, but to recognize them as human. Such realizations generate an understanding of these self-motivated patterns, which can be used to create new habituated responses that are less selfish. The Ch'an

Buddhism objective is to reach a point of calmness and acceptance where words, deeds, and thoughts are beyond reproach; in Taoism, the goal is Wu Wei, regrettable necessity, where the individual acts in accord with nature and ethics. Ultimately, self-interest may be impossible to eradicate entirely, but the purpose is to speak and act with greater self-awareness, and in adjusting one's responses, an individual removes emotional and psychological obstacles to the cultivation of the self.

Life Applications

Learning fighting applications is central to training in the Internal Martial Arts, but it is equally important to apply to life the principles of Qi, Jing, and Shen. A vital and necessary part of daily practice is self-assessment and reflection. (See Table 1.1 for an overview of how this practice relates to the energy equation discussed in Chapter 1.)

Some of these inputs and outputs we have control over such as what we eat, how much we sleep, who we spend free time with, what kind of relationships we have, and what forms of exercise and activities we do. Other things we do not have such control over such as environmental pollutants, work environments and coworkers, and tasks that must be addressed.

A number of questions can help to direct assessment:

- Is this a good use of my time and energy?

- Is this relationship beneficial?

- How does eating this particular food make me feel?

- How do I feel after spending my time doing (a particular task, a form of exercise, and so forth)?

- What changes can be made?

An assessment of these things should be a regular part of life so as to better understand the state of mind, health, and well-being, and how that state is an extension of these other factors. Limiting our exposure to environments, people, and relationships that are detrimental to ourselves is vital, and recognition of those negative things is a necessary condition to be able to make changes. While we may not have control to change negative outputs completely, our insights may be useful in making slight adjustments that minimize or lessen the impact of any negative outputs. As Dr. Yang once remarked during a seminar on medical and therapeutic Qigong, the bottom line to being healthy is "Find out what is bothering you, and fix it."

We must train to transform negative emotions, stress, and anxiety into positive emotions and a calm mental state. Transforming ourselves begins with our choices—what we eat, what we do, and with whom we spend time—but it also means that we must be aware of our habituated emotional responses to experiences, obstacles, and events of our day-to-day life. When we become aware of the negative outputs in our life, we identify the issues, relationships, and things that we need to address and change. As we train the mind to be more self-aware, this leads to the ability to alter the ways in which we interact with the external world, thereby providing the key to make a direct impact upon environment, social situations, and work.

The Principle of Training

Since energy, vitality, and spirit are inextricably intertwined, training requires paying attention to body, breath, mind, and energy. To only do physical exercise without self-reflection would be like only lifting weights with one arm. Similarly, to meditate without proper energy work would be repeating the mistakes of the monks that Bodhidharma first encountered when he arrived at the Shaolin monastery: they lacked sufficient energy to sustain their meditative practice. Training should be approached with the principle of being humanly complete and unified, and each of these training techniques is designed to enhance the others. While each facet of training is separate, they are all tools on the path toward a unified, whole self. These various training facets function like the process of the Five Elements Theory where each nurtures, generates, and balances the others in an ongoing cycle of harmonization and cultivation.

Coda

Master Jou (Tsung Hwa) would often repeat four basic rules for practice of the Internal Arts, and those rules are invaluable in approaching the essence of training in energy, vitality, and spirit:

1. Know yourself.

2. Do your best.

3. Don't overdo it.

4. Every day make yourself better.

The way of energy, vitality, and spirit is a unified approach in the pursuit of understanding the self, striving for excellence and balance, and becoming a better human being. That cultivation is progression toward being a more fully realized person at peace and tranquil internally and in the world. The path of being such a person—what Taoism calls a "Real Human" and a sage—is to engage in the continuous process of navigating the ebb and flow of Qi, and tracing the way to the Source in order to nurture the Qi of life.

Endnotes

1. See Chapter 3 for illustrations of the energetic and organ channels of the body.

2. If a person experiences cool Yin Qi, it is recommended to contact a Traditional Chinese Medicine doctor, since such feeling may indicate an imbalance in the body that needs to be adjusted.

3. Holding the breath can be harmful and is not recommended for extended practice.

4. See the "Standing Pole Qigong" discussion in Chapter 6 for a detailed discussion of this stance.

5. The Microcosmic Orbit is an Inner Alchemical Taoist technique used to circulate the Qi from the Dantian and up the Governing Channel of the back and then down the Conception Channel of the front of the body. The Microcosmic Orbit is sometimes called the Small Circuit and this pathway forms the connected loop of the Governing and Conception channels. The meditative technique of Microcosmic Breathing or Meditation is one of actively leading Qi through this circuit.

6. The process of converting Qi to Jin is touched upon later in this chapter.

7. The Eight Extraordinary Channels are more detailed and expansive, and it is not within the purview of this study to offer anything more than a basic sketch of these channels. If the reader wishes to explore this information in much greater detail, I recommend a course of study that addresses the specifics of Traditional Chinese Medicine. Dr. Yang's *The Root of Chinese Qigong: Secrets for Health, Longevity, and Enlightenment* (Yang 1989) is an excellent starting point.

8. Ted Kaptchuk's classic *The Web That Has No Weaver: Understanding Chinese Medicine* (Kaptchuk 1983) offers an excellent introduction to the methodologies and the diagnostic practices related to the Organ Channels.

9. For bow stance, the back foot toes turn slightly outward at approximately thirty-five degrees. The toes of the front foot are straight facing forward. The weight is 60 percent forward and 40 percent back, and the feet are shoulder width.

10. Master Sun Lu Tang—famous for his Hsing-I and Bagua and the creator of Sun-style Taiji—placed great importance on this position and referred to this as "San Ti." Similarly, according to Master Yang Yang, Chen-style Taiji values this meditative stance highly and often refers to this posture as a closed secret that is absolutely vital in training in Chen style.

11. This stance is also employed for general circle walking in many styles of Baguazhang.

12. These energies are referred to as Peng, Lu, Ji, An, Cai, Lieh, Zhou, and Khou, or Ward-off, Roll-back, Squeeze, Press (downward), Pluck, Split, Elbow Strike, and Shoulder Strike.

13. Traditional Qigong training refers to these methods as the "three adjustments of body, breath, and mind," which are the foundation for developing Qigong gong fa (or forms).

14. *Breath in Action: the Art of Breath in Vocal and Holistic Practices*, edited by Jane Boston and Nena Cook (London: Jessica Kingsley Publishers, 2009), provides an excellent overview of breathing strategies and health. The focus here is not to cover all of the health benefits of proper breathing, especially since other students have already done that quite well. My purpose is to link the discussion of breathing with the realm of Traditional Chinese Medicine and the life of Qi.

15. Even fewer people, according to Dr. Yang, are able to direct Qi, and it is extremely rare that a person can regulate Shen (spirit). This book is my response to the challenge of the difficulty of regulating Qi and Shen, and presents principles and methods to help others learn how to regulate Qi and, in this chapter, how that Qi transforms into Shen.

16. This is not to suggest that in order to be healthy all emotions are to be eliminated. Again, such a misinterpretation has grown out of the misperception that so-called masters of Buddhism, Taoism, and Internal Arts are apathetic. Calmness and tranquility in the face of adversity is mistaken for apathy.

17. See Chapter 6 for a detailed explanation of how to do this meditation as a seated exercise.

18. The proper technique for Embryonic Breathing is extremely complex, and as a form of meditative Qigong it is well beyond the scope of this book. Anyone wishing to read more about the philosophy and technique of Embryonic Breathing is urged to consult *Qigong Meditation: Embryonic Breathing*, Yang (2003). Furthermore, anyone wishing to try this technique should work closely with an experienced teacher. This is not a technique that should be approached without expert guidance. As the famous Taoist Ancestor Lu warns, "Once you have made the great elixir, essence and sense submit, and the earthly and celestial are in their places. It is necessary, however, to seek elevated Real People to indicate to you the hidden subtleties in order that the proper results be attained" (Cleary 1991a, p.81).

References

Boston, J. and Cook, R. (eds) (2009) *Breath in Action: The Art of Breath in Vocal and Holistic Practice.* London: Jessica Kingsley Publishers.

Byrom, T. (1993) *Dhammapada: The Sayings of the Buddha.* Boston, MA: Shambhala.

Cleary, T. (1991a) *Vitality, Energy, Spirit: A Taoist Sourcebook.* Boston, MA: Shambhala.

Cleary, T. (1991b) *The Secret of the Golden Flower: The Classic Chinese Book of Life.* New York, NY: Harper.

Cleary, T. (1992) *The Essential Tao.* San Francisco, CA: Castle Books.

Cleary, T. (1996) *Practical Taoism.* Boston, MA: Shambhala.

Cleary, T. (2000) *Taoist Meditation: Methods for Cultivating a Healthy Mind and Body.* Boston, MA: Shambhala.

Cleary, T. (2003a) *The Taoist Classics. Volume One.* Boston, MA: Shambhala.

Cleary, T. (2003b) *The Taoist Classics. Volume Two.* Boston, MA: Shambhala.

Cleary, T. (2003c) *The Taoist Classics. Volume Three.* Boston, MA: Shambhala.

Deng, M. (1996) *Everyday Tao: Living with Balance and Harmony.* New York, NY: Harper.

Erdman, D.V. (ed.) (1988) "The Marriage of Heaven and Hell." In *The Complete Poetry and Prose of William Blake: Newly Revised Edition.* New York, NY: Doubleday.

Kaptchuk, T. (1983) *The Web That Has No Weaver: Understanding Chinese Medicine.* New York, NY: Congdon and Weed.

Kohn, L. (2008) *Chinese Healing Exercises: The Tradition of Daoyin.* Honolulu, HI: University of Hawai'i Press.

Miller, D. (ed.) (1993) *Xing Yi Quan Xue: The Study of Form-Mind Boxing.* Dallas, TX: Beckett Media.

Mitchell, S. (ed.) (1989) "Archaic Torso of Apollo" in *The Selected Poetry of Rainer Maria Rilke.* New York, NY: Vintage.

Ni, M. (1995) *The Yellow Emperor's Classic of Medicine.* Boston, MA: Shambhala.

Pine, R. (1987) *The Zen Teaching of Bodhidharma.* New York, NY: North Point Press.

Sayre, R.F. (ed.) (1985) *Thoreau.* New York, NY: Library of America.

Wile, D. (1983) *T'ai-chi Touchstones: Yang Family Secret Transmissions.* Brooklyn, NY: Sweet Chi Press.

Yang, J. (1989) *The Root of Chinese Qigong: Secrets for Health, Longevity, and Enlightenment.* Roslindale, MA: YMAA Publishing.

Yang, J. (2003) *Qigong Meditation: Embryonic Breathing.* Roslindale, MA: YMAA Publishing.

Yu, A. (2006) *The Monkey and the Monk: An Abridgment of The Journey to the West.* Chicago, IL: University of Chicago Press.